# SURVIVING MENTAL ILLNESS THROUGH HUMOR

A collection of essays showcasing the hopes, despair, and hilarity of writers on their personal journey with Mental Illness.

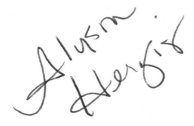

*Alyson Herzig and Jessica Azar*

Surviving Mental Illness Through Humor

Cover design by Marta Chade

*This book is dedicated to every person who has ever struggled with a mental illness; together we can end the stigma.*

I would like to thank my husband John and our children, Jacob and Jillian, for their patience and support during my journey to see this project to fruition. ~ Alyson Herzig

Thank you, God, for blessing me with both the challenges and talents needed to complete this project. Zack, thank you for supporting me on this journey and loving me through the highs and lows of the illness that led to the creation of this book. ZV, Ben, Mary Ellen and Bebe, I love you. ~ Jessica Azar

Here is what people are saying about Surviving Mental Illness Through Humor:

"You should totally buy this book." ~ Jenny Lawson, New York Times Bestselling Author of *Let's Pretend This Never Happened*

"A much needed compilation that opens the dialogue on Mental Illness and helps fight stigma." ~ Robin O'Bryant, New York Times Bestselling Author of *Ketchup is a Vegetable: And Other Lies Moms Tell Themselves*

"To be brave is to be afraid and push through that fear. The essays in this anthology epitomize courage." ~ Sarah Fader, Creator and CEO of StigmaFighters

"Books like this are desperately needed to offer hope to those who deal with mental illness—and enlighten those who don't. Filled with brave and insightful stories, this anthology is an important contribution to the movement to end the stigma of mental illness." ~ J.D. Bailey, Creator of Honest Mom®

# TABLE OF CONTENTS

# FOREWORD
## Nicole Knepper

When meeting new people, it's not uncommon to break the ice with a conversation about jobs. Work tends to be a safe subject that leads to other benign, surface topics, and keeps the chit-chat chugging along comfortably. I am always hesitant to fully answer this question, even though it's a totally appropriate inquiry. Usually, I say that I'm a writer, and then when asked what I write about, I tell them that it's mostly technical stuff for porn websites. That statement either awkwardly ends the discussion or pulverizes the ice into warm giggles. The only time I share that I am a clinical psychotherapist, as well as a writer, is if there's a delicious seafood buffet. My disclosure opens the door to the complicated subject of mental health, and gets people talking.

The more they talk, the less they eat, which means more shrimp and imitation crab meat for me!

"So I have a friend who…" or "Can I get your professional opinion about…" or, "I once had a therapist …" and every so often I get, "Can you write me a prescription for Xanax?" and of course I say yes, but I let them know that because I'm not a medical doctor, the pharmacy probably won't fill the prescription.

Sometimes that successfully ends the conversation. Sometimes not.

Occasionally people will unload a stream of consciousness full of awkward, intimate, painful, or hilarious anecdotes about their mental health related adventures with something or someone.

Other times they say:

"Isn't your job just SO depressing?"

"Don't you get tired of listening to people whine?"

When I'm asked *those* questions, I simply respond with a question of my own:

"Will you tell me why you think I would feel that way about my job?"

Then they do... they always do. People are fascinating and complicated. I soak up their verbal and emotional chaos as I shove seafood into my gob at warp speed. I've learned that answering a question with a question is brilliant strategy at social gatherings in warm weather, because shrimp is so much tastier when it's still nice and chilled. I like my shrimp chilled. So, while people are telling me about their mom (It's always the mom), I listen.

That's what I do, you know? I am a professional listener.

When the shrimp is gone and I have listened to endless stories about horrible mothers, I address their original question, because I cannot let anyone think anything negative about my life's work for one second after the last shrimp hits my belly! NO!

I tell them that being a clinical therapist is NOT depressing. Not one bit!

I tell them that it's a hopeful and positive job and how much I love it.

I tell them that I feel privileged to be trusted with sacred, private thoughts and secrets, to act as a collaborator, using my best self to tease out the best self of my clients as they learn and grow and heal.

I tell them that I never, EVER get tired of listening to people whine, because that's not what people are doing when they come to therapy. Streams of consciousness aren't complaints and criticisms! The words shared in session are full of feelings and ideas needing to be refined, clarified, understood, and accepted. I talk a little and I listen a lot. I reflect, support, educate, and validate as the people I work with reveal the strength and hope that brought them to therapy in the first place.

This is a book full of stories written by people that are hopeful, strong, and brave enough to talk about their mental health struggles. By breaking the silence with their honest stories, they give others hope, help normalize mental illness and the struggle, and crush the stigma that is still acting as a cloak of shame worn by those who are still suffering in silence.

Mental illness is not a choice! It's not a weakness of character, or something a person can will away or have shamed out of them, as so many people incorrectly still believe. Too many!

This. Has. To. Stop! Talking about mental illness, honestly, openly, bravely, and loudly is how we start the stopping! Start stopping stigma! Say that five times fast. You can say it and you can do it.

YOU CAN! WE CAN! AND WE MUST!

The ignorance, fear, the devastating guilt and shame people surrounding mental illness have no place in a world where we have the tools, technology, and knowledge to treat them. Many mental health conditions are as common and manageable as are so many other physical health conditions.

Yes, mental illness is a health condition. And more. So very much more.

As Kimberly Morand, one of the contributors to this anthology, so perfectly described, people with mental illnesses are simply, "a giant mish-mosh of sucky genes, chemistry, and circumstances." I hope you enjoy reading this mish-mosh amazing authors and their stories. I hope you share it, talk about it, and start the stopping of mental health stigma. That's what we are doing here. One story at a time.

*Nicole Knepper is a licensed clinical professional counselor, author, blogger and social media addict. Her <u>Moms Who Drink And Swear Facebook</u> community inspired her blog and best-selling book. In a perfect world, she would not be asked to explain why she doesn't use her gigantic platform as a conduit for cash and celebrity, but the world is not perfect, so when asked why she blows so many opportunities to achieve the fame and fortune so many other bloggers crave, she engages in stonewalling and writes blog posts with bad words about random topics - like porn and poetry.*

# INTRODUCTION

The vase slipped through my hands and crashed to the floor, shattering into pieces. I stood frozen looking down at the destruction, unsure which way to step. The wrong move would result in a deep cut, the only option was to take a large ungraceful step and pray I didn't land on a sharp edge. I didn't have time for this today, though there never is a good time, is there?

Frustrated and angry, I bent down and picked up the shards of glass. They were scattered into the far corners of my kitchen, hidden under the cabinets, lying in wait for days or weeks until I would unexpectedly step on one. The pain would sear through my limb, the annoyance at having again failed at a task. I could scream. But I won't scream. I will fight back the tears, the hurt, the anger, and move on. Because this is what I do, I compartmentalize my emotions.

My life is a lot like the vase that broke into a million fragments. For so long it was beautiful, held together perfectly. Created by the hands of another. It had purpose. There was a reason for it. But then it shattered, in one moment. There had been cracks for years, but I ignored them. As much as I wanted to paint a picture of my strength and capability, the reality is I was one fumble from disaster. I had spent decades of my life filing the anger, embarrassment, pain, and hatred into the back recesses of my mind until there were no corners left to hide the thoughts in.

The anxiety and panic came in pounding waves. I lay in a fetal position unable to breathe. Each breath was painful and worse than the one before. My mind had betrayed me. I had worked so hard to bury the worry because I was told I had to, there was no choice. I had kept all the pain inside. Years of hyper-awareness and no one to confide in left my psyche fragile. I felt so alone. Who would understand? If I began to peel back my armor and show myself would anyone be there to hold me? To help me? Was I just being weak?

At thirty-eight years old I finally took down my shield and shared my story on my personal blog. Maybe it would help people realize I am not who they thought I was, that my shyness is based upon my own insecurities. Part of me wanted to explain my actions to those who know me and had been near me when my panic and anxiety took over. I felt I owed it to them and I owed it to myself.

The first person to contact me after I shared my story is the co-creator of this anthology, Jessica Azar. We did not know each other before, but were introduced through the wonderment of social media. She shared with me her personal struggles with her own illness, bipolar. I no longer felt so alone. Someone else understood my issues and offered me a shoulder to lean on. Jessica and I have forged a tight bond and invite you to join us in our quest to destigmatize mental illness.

We hope that, as you read this book, you will realize you are not alone. In the pages of this book you will find others who have shared the same feelings of worthlessness, exhaustion, anger, and loneliness. You will read their words and understand how they saw suicide not as an end, but as a way to save those who love them more than they could love themselves. I hope you find solace in realizing there is help, and you are more than the sum of your actions.

Unlike any other book you will pick up about mental illness, you will also find humor amongst these pages. You will smile, nod, chuckle, and laugh out loud at the stories of others, like you, have shared. As you know, mental illness is not all just lows. There are moments of laughter sprinkled in. It is the ability to find the funny in the times we don't expect it that will help you become whole again. We have woven the humor pieces amongst the mental illness essays in a manner that mimics life. You may go from the high of laughing at the unfortunate circumstances of one writer, to feeling the deep pain and heartache of another. This is life, the ups and the downs.

Just like the broken vase, there are many fragments to us. Individually they are useless, but when you take the time to glue them together you may find a new beauty and purpose. Thank you for taking the time to turn these pages, and may you find comfort in knowing you are not alone. All of the authors have selected a local charity in their communities whose purpose is to help others with mental illness. Our goal is to pay it forward, because every person is worth it.

Alyson Herzig

# VOLUNTARY ADMISSION
## Kimberly Morand

The rain fell outside my window. Ominous clouds suffocated the skyline, fusing together the world's brilliant colors of promise and the lifeless shades of melancholia. Autumn's chill was in each violent gust of wind that lifted the frayed edges of our patio screen. I pulled my scarf up to my chin and grabbed for my cup of tea, which had long gone cold. The soft, lamenting music that meandered throughout the kitchen grabbed hold of my soul and danced with my hopelessness. My legs were frozen with numbness from sitting in the same spot for what seemed like an eternity; I was unable to move forward with my life or death. No written words from my aching soul touched the blank page that lay before me, but it was marred with the pain that was encapsulated in each tear drop that fell upon it. I was preparing my letter to explain, to help, to offer insight, to say good-bye. I was planning my suicide.

Much like a malcontented salesman is excited by daydreams of winning the lottery, the fleeting thoughts of suicide excited me. I was conscious of all the practical dangers that could provide convincing opportunities for deliberate "accidents," like holding my wrist in the way of a sharp knife as it cut through a watermelon, or swerving my car into a light pole. I balanced myself on curbsides as cars approached from behind and imagined what it would be like if I just stepped off, pretending to fall onto the street and turn toward the noise. There would be no commotion as the car forced its way through my unyielding pain. Hundreds of moments would meld into one life, my life, as my feet lifted off of the ground. Suicidal thoughts would fly on soft wisps of wind that tickled the trees as the car's impact ripped my soul from my body.

Peace.

These thoughts gave me a rush that no drug could ever replicate and I became fixated on them. I replayed them like a newly discovered song, trying to figure out the lyrics and then belting them out in perfect harmony. My soul's misery was co-writing my swan song with my brain's creativity.

"Are we going for a drive today?" my son asked, startling me out of my bleak thoughts. The freezing, early-morning temperatures would have normally deterred me but for some reason I was compelled to walk him to school that day.

"Let's walk today, buddy. I need some fresh air," I said as I grabbed my coat and his hat.

Despite the early hour our neighborhood was oddly alive. We heard the sounds of dead twigs ricocheting off metal before they were shot out the side of lawnmowers and the crunching of weightless leaves as they were forced into yard waste bags. Parents were shouting as they chased after their boisterous kids with forgotten lunch bags, followed by the heavy breath of a runner who passed by us and the sound of my son's zealous voice trying to push through it all.

We shuffled through the fallen leaves that converged at the school's entrance. "This is how you do it," my son said as if he were the master of leaf kicks. He was only four years old, but was already a great teacher of finding joy in the little things. I smiled weakly at him, but didn't respond. Before I let his hand go, he grabbed a hold of my leg and said quietly, "Momma, you look so beautiful today. I am proud of you." His words cut through my death-occupied reverie like a breath of air in empty lungs. Part of me awakened enough to know that I didn't want to die. That afternoon, I voluntarily admitted myself to the hospital.

Three hundred ninety two. That's the number of slats in the air vents under the window. A small amount of glitter was peppered where the vent met the tile on the floor. I mustered up a weak giggle, thinking of the irony in something so readily associated with magical happiness and unicorns somehow finding its way into this room. A pipe dream. I gathered up the edges of the worn blankets laced with the smell of disinfectant and curled myself into a protective ball on the uncomfortably concave mattress. I began to think about the woman who had occupied my bed hours before I "moved in." I wondered if she had found herself. I imagined her smile as she walked out the locked doors and into the sun. I was both jealous and happy for her, and yearned to be well enough to do the same as I drifted off to sleep.

It startled me when the nurse intentionally bumped the side of my bed to wake me up. As I tried to remember where I was and how I had gotten there, she introduced herself and then she handed me two sheets of blank paper and a mini pencil.

"I want you to write about what brought you here and what emotions you are experiencing. Write about what worries you or makes you feel those intense emotions that provoke you to hurt yourself. We will meet later to go over your notes. We'll discuss this and form a plan of care," she said.

It took me three hours to write the four words: *I am so sorry.*

I thought of that morning and got sick to my stomach as I looked at those words. I folded that paper until it was tiny enough to hide in the trashcan, mirroring the smallness I felt internally.

The nurses kicked me out of my room after I had spent most of the day huddled in my new "home." I reclaimed my solitude on a wooden bench that spanned half of the corridor. I liked this spot on the ward, or the "Puzzle Factory," as the other patients called it. "Everyone is trying to find the missing pieces to their happiness and sanity," a patient told me. I watched the other patients roam the hallways as they made a left, then another left, and then another, until they had completed the circle. It wasn't a race or for exercise; it was merely something to occupy the time while hoping that clarity of mind would present itself.

Whenever one of us encountered someone new on the hall, we introduced ourselves with one simple question. "Whatcha in for?"

The answers ran the gamut: psychosis, bipolar disorder, depression, and schizophrenia. We were a giant mish-mosh of sucky genes, chemistry, and circumstance. I was fascinated with everyone's stories. It didn't matter who they were or how they got there, we shared a pain so deep that none of the people waiting for us outside of those walls could ever understand. Despite our connection through mental illness, however, I realized I missed my family, the very ones I was going to leave behind, whether they fully understood the depths of my sorrow or not.

I wandered back to my room and sat on the bed, thinking about the long road of healing that lay before me, when I heard a soft tap on my door.

"I love what you've done to the place. It's very homey," my husband Shawn said, breaking up the silence as he entered my room. He kissed my forehead sweetly and I pulled him in closer so the scent of his aftershave would stay with me when I slept. He brought heaven in a coffee cup and the world to me in stories.

"So we didn't have lunch meat and I had to improvise. I sent the kid to school with a jelly sandwich, but I can't remember if I put him in socks because he didn't come home wearing any. He did come home in the same underwear I sent him to school with, but they were from yesterday. My Father's Day card is going to suck this year isn't it?" he joked.

I was entranced by his facial features and every gesture he made. If I had gone through with my plan I would have left my pain behind for him to bear. The thought of never again sharing the love that intertwined two souls who dreamed big, of never again sharing laughter, of never again feeling his embrace that made me feel so safe, of never attaining our future goal of becoming laxative drug lords in a nursing home together. I would have lost it all and I would have stolen those same things from him.

A nurse passed by the room and barked, "He can't be in here."

Shawn stood and said, "I have to go anyway. Uncle Jeff probably threw a blanket over Chase's head with the hopes of making him disappear. That kid is hopped up on his jelly sandwich and the gummy worms I gave him. I feel bad for Jeff. I feel bad for you," he said as I heard his voice crack. "Get better okay? I need you. I love you."

That night I slept with my shirt pulled over my nose to breathe him in. His scent kept me comforted for the remainder of the time I was there.

Mondays were discharge days. I had been there for five long days and a scuffle with a violent patient had scared me enough to expedite my desire to go home. During my evaluation with the psychiatrist, he apologized for the incident.

"I'm so sorry for what happened with the other patient," my psychiatrist said, as a charge nurse jotted down notes.

"Well I guess that I can scratch 'getting punched in the face for stabbing someone with an imaginary knife' off of my bucket list," I joked.

"How are you feeling? Are you having any thoughts of hurting yourself or suicide, Kim?" he asked. My answer was interrupted when my roommate burst into the room and started off on a tangent. While the doctor tried to calm my roommate, I looked over his shoulder and eyed the tall antenna tower on another building. I had frequently stared at it when I was in bed for the first couple of days. I had thought about climbing it and diving off it over and over and over. I shuddered. Those thoughts were no longer clawing at my mind.

After my roommate has been quieted and sent away, the psychiatrist sat back down and looked at me.

"Do you want to go home?" Dr. B asked.

I nodded my head yes. I wanted to go home.

My senses were overwhelmed when the soles of my boots hit the pavement outside the hospital. The sun was so bright that it was almost painful and the slightest noise seemed amplified. I imagined that this must be exactly how a newborn feels: overwhelmed by the newness of it all and trying to find some safe arms to land into. I suppose that leaving the psychiatric ward is like a rebirth of sorts. I was re-entering the world of everyday life as abruptly as I had left it.

When I got home, I was tackled by my dog's joyful ninety pounds of pure ignorance. I flapped his soft ears and kissed his head. "It smells like a jock strap in here," I said as I stood up. The floors were unswept and peppered with building blocks. There were dishes in the sink growing ungodly things. The bathroom was littered with towels and mini underwear. The beds were unmade. Our home was a complete disaster, but it could be fixed. Hopefulness that everything in our lives could be repaired surrounded me.

"So I couldn't find the dishwasher but will you look at that, she's standing in the kitchen right now!" Shawn joked.

"Momma!" my son said as he plowed into my legs, knocking me off kilter. "I missed you for all of the days." I brushed my hand over the top of his head. The thought of never again seeing his face, of never again feeling those chubby arms tightly wrapped around my neck as his face pressed into my shoulder, of never being a witness to where his feet will take him in his life. The idea of never being a part of that adventure pierced my soul in a way that was previously unimaginable to me.

Amidst the chaos in my head, I found my purpose in their smiles.

Today, the rain falls outside my window and my tea has gone cold; it's eerily reminiscent of that day. It's been three years since my hospital admission. It's not an anniversary that anyone would want to mark on a calendar or buy a cake to celebrate. I don't know how I should feel about it, or if I'm supposed to feel anything at all. I've made it this far, and that is worth celebrating.

I do know that I need to be here for them and for myself. And for now, that's enough.

*Kimberly Morand is a mom, wife, nurse, mental health advocate, and full time chocolate hater. When she's not busy pretending to look busy, she's writing for* SZ Magazine, Anchor: Conquering Depression, Bipolar and Anxiety. *Her work can also be found in the books* Clash Of The Couples *and* The Good Mother Myth: Redefining Motherhood to Fit Reality. *Kimberly was the first Canadian member to join the talented cast of the 2014* Listen To Your Mother Show: Metro Detroit. *She fears spiders, public restrooms, and your mom's cooking.*

# THE WALLS CAME TUMBLING DOWN

## Kathleen Gordon

All my life I've been what you'd call tightly wound. I sweat the small stuff. On bad days, I feel vulnerable and exposed, like I'm walking around with no skin. If I were a car, I would have no shock absorbers, and every pothole, every pebble, would feel like an assault. I'm easily overwhelmed by things that just don't seem to faze other people. Those frustrating days everyone has when everything seems to go wrong, can completely derail me if I'm not careful. I hate to feel like I'm disappointing people and I fear that if anyone knew what a mess I am inside, they'd reject me. Sometimes, when things are particularly bad, I shut down in panic. It took me nearly four decades to realize this is not normal.

Some of my family members have significant mental health issues, but they did not have the resources or insight to address them effectively while I was growing up. My middle class childhood looked fine from the outside, but behind closed doors, it was unstable and chaotic. I never knew how people in my house were going to behave under that day's circumstances, and the emotional atmosphere at any time was subject to change without notice. I didn't feel safe expressing my feelings or opinions. There was a lot of pressure on me to not be a problem, to maintain the status quo, to be a good girl. Aside from some minor teen rebellion, I did as I was told. I spent my high school and college years working to get out of my hometown, thinking that would solve things, but I neglected to realize that I couldn't leave myself behind and that my problems would travel with me.

In 2007, I was the stay-home mother of a two-year-old daughter and a "spirited" four-year-old son (later diagnosed with autism/Asperger's disorder). I discovered that I was not a good fit for the isolation of endlessly tending to and cleaning up after demanding short people, beloved though they were to me. I did not have any emotional or practical support from my then-husband, in part because I was not good at asking for it. I had been picking up a little part time work to preserve career options for later, when the kids were older, but I discovered that the amount of logistical prep required to make that happen was tantamount to having a full time job, minus paid sick leave or benefits. Each day, I felt like I was barely keeping myself together with chewing gum and baling wire, hanging on with white knuckles, waiting for it all to come crashing apart.

As the year careened to a close and the holidays approached, I could feel my internal tension ratcheting up. I couldn't sleep well, and each morning it was harder to drag myself out of bed. I was tearful, though I couldn't articulate why. Every little setback felt traumatic and the hits just kept on coming. It was the emotional equivalent of wearing a coarse, itchy wool bodysuit over bare skin on a hot day, and I couldn't take it off. Worst of all, it felt like nobody noticed or cared, although I was too afraid to tell anyone outright. When I finally I tried to explain things to my husband, he told me I just needed to relax, that everything would be okay. He meant well, but he might as well have been telling me to sprout wings and fly. I was at my breaking point.

Our plan was to take a holiday road trip to visit both sides of the family. The day we planned to leave, I drove to pick up my children from preschool and we needed to get on the road immediately afterward. I remember a litany of worries flying at me like bricks. Would the kids be at least somewhat well-behaved? Would my parents judge my parenting because my son seemed to be having issues we did not yet understand? Would they make it worse, as they generally did? Would I have any chance at a break? Would I ever get a break from this feeling of impending doom, or would it just go on forever until I died? I felt light-headed and realized I was hyperventilating. For a moment, I wondered what would happen if I pointed the car in any direction and just kept driving, not telling anyone where I had gone. Then I wondered what would happen if I plowed the car into a telephone pole. Maybe everyone would be better off, and at least I wouldn't have to live like this anymore.

That thought stopped me cold and I pulled over. I knew that I could not put my children in the car unless I could pull myself together. It took a very long time. I cried. I screamed. I swore. I felt like I was in a dark tunnel, trying to claw my way back to the surface. When I finally exhausted myself, I breathed deeply until my vision returned to normal and I could hear my phone buzzing at me over the pounding in my ears. It was the preschool, telling me I was late for pickup, again. I apologized and said I was stuck in traffic. The director asked me if I was all right. I lied and said I was, but I don't think I was fooling anyone. I drove to a fast food place and splashed cold water on my face in the restroom, looked in the mirror, and reassured myself that I was not going to lose my damn mind that day.

I'd like to say I immediately got help, that the people around me understood what I needed, and that we all lived happily ever after. I didn't, they didn't, and we didn't.

We took that trip to see our families as planned. The last place I needed to be was in the house where I grew up, and it was every bit as awful as I'd feared. I had a panic attack in my parents' house, in the bathroom with the water running, and another panic attack when we got home, this time in front of my husband, who told me "for Christ's sake get a grip!" I responded by curling more tightly into the fetal position on the shower floor and whimpering; spots swam before my eyes. Although I never had outright suicidal intentions, and I didn't actually want to die, I wasn't sure how much more I could take before my brain broke. I was hanging onto my sanity by my fingernails.

Eventually, thankfully, I stumbled into therapy. I was diagnosed with an anxiety disorder and my doctor said it was no wonder I was having a breakdown. He was, quite frankly, amazed it hadn't happened years earlier, and he observed that my ability to avoid completely losing my shit until I was almost forty was a testament to my inner strength. I'd never thought of it that way before; it was enlightening. I started taking antidepressant medications that, after a while, started to help me feel better. It didn't happen overnight and it didn't happen on a steady trajectory. I had to make some difficult decisions, which included getting a divorce and going back to work full time. There were good days and bad days, but I held on. One morning, as I drove to work, I thought to myself, "Holy crap! This is how most people get to feel every day!"

By virtue of brain chemistry, I will probably always run a bit hot, but I am developing better ways of managing it. I avoid putting myself in situations that trigger my anxiety. I try to take good care of myself physically so that I have the resources I need to control my emotions instead of letting them control me. I have a script for dealing with times of panic so that I don't end up on the edge like I did before. I set boundaries with other people and tell them what I will and won't do, knowing that their reactions are their problem, not mine.

All of this has helped me have a life I hadn't thought possible seven years ago. I am a much better mother now that I'm not merely trying to survive. Both of my children are thriving. I enjoy my job, and I've thrown myself into writing as a creative outlet. I'm invested in my friendships. I have an attentive, loving boyfriend. Best of all, I see life again as something to be enjoyed rather than endured.

If I could go back and speak to myself during that dark time, I would tell myself not to wait so long to seek help, and that admitting defeat is sometimes the strongest thing you can do. I would remind myself that I was worth saving, both on my own account as well as on behalf of my children and everyone else who loves me. These are the same things I would say to anyone going through a dark place. You are enough. You are worthwhile. You do not need to suffer alone.

*Kathleen Gordon is a lawyer with a dirty mind who uses inappropriate humor as a defense mechanism. She's also a single mom of two children, Tweak (10) and Tink (8). She began writing on her blog,* Middletini, *to process her feelings about heading into her 40s, nearly losing her damn mind because her life had not turned out as planned, and getting her groove back with a little help from her friends and the occasional adult beverage. Each post opens with a suggested cocktail, because she's less offensive when you've been drinking. Kathleen likes to write about the things people think to themselves but have the common sense not to say out loud. She is writing a novel in her abundant spare time.*

# WAITING FOR THE MILK CART

## Sherry Vondy Beaver

W hen my father was in the mental hospital he sewed mocca-sins from kits and glued turquoise and orange tiles into ash-tray molds. Such was therapy in the 1960s. I was five. My biggest worry was what to take to Show and Tell the following week; my mother gave me a resounding "no" when I asked to take one of Dad's creations.

We lived in a tiny town in northeastern Colorado. Feedlots to the north and west, beef packing plant to the south. No matter where you went, cattle were putting in their two cents. With a population of only 8,000, there was always a feeling that everyone always knew your business.

Having my father's anxiety-making genes, my own anxiety rose as I contemplated my upcoming turn at public speaking. I'd put it off as long as I could and now the teacher was pressuring me. "Looks like the only person we haven't heard from lately is ... Sherry."

Unfortunately, I'd already exhausted my cache of things to show. Paper doll sets. A prized marble. The scar on my hand from where I fell on a glass bottle of bubbles. There was no way around it, I'd have to come up with a "tell." Quick. But what?

Aside from an occasional ride-along to the grocery store or downtown, I'd never been anywhere interesting. My older sister's life of junior high homework and boys seemed boring. No worthy stories there. And, even though Mom got excited talking about how hard it was to pay bills, I was pretty sure that topic was off limits.

Then, it happened. A miracle. My mother announced that we were going to Denver to see my dad. Denver. The big city. A place I'd heard about but never dreamed I'd go. On Saturday, we piled into the Rambler and drove two hundred miles through country so brown and desolate the only scenery was the occasional tumbleweed blowing across the road at 30 miles an hour.

The highlights of the trip were staying in a motel, ordering hamburgers from a drive-thru window, and going to see my dad in the hospital. He showed me one of the moccasin kits, how to thread the leather cord through the pre-punched holes of the sole. I even got to sew a little bit on one of them. "Let the other kids top that," I thought. I was ready for Show and Tell.

All day Monday my heart raced; it landed in my throat when the moment came, beating so hard I thought it might leap outside my body. My fellow kindergartners sat on the floor, picking their noses, squirming with boredom, or dwelling on their own imminent turns in the spotlight. I walked to the front of the room, fearing I would pass out, unable to breathe. Courageously, I stepped up on the chair and addressed my audience.

"I went to Denver and saw my dad," I blurted. Anything else stumbling out of my mouth, beyond that statement, is a mystery to this day. From the moment I took the stage the focus was on the exit. When it was over, relief turned to joy and confidence. Victory.

As usual, my mother waited in the car after school, parked along the curb in the same spot. I raced toward her with pride, knowing she would be amazed by my pluck. Perhaps ice cream would be served in my honor at dinner that night. Maybe she would call her friends to brag. I climbed in the passenger seat and shared my accomplishment.

"Oh, my god," she said. "You told them what?"

"I told them we saw Dad."

"Oh, god. Did you tell them which hospital he's in?"

"I don't know. Maybe."

"Oh, god. I don't want kids going home and telling their parents."

This was not the reaction I anticipated. Obviously I had done something horribly wrong. My previous satisfaction quickly melted into hot sticky shame. "Listen," she said. "You have to go back up there tomorrow. You have to tell them your father's in the hospital because he hurt his back."

His back?

I had no idea why my father was hospitalized, but a back injury sounded fishy. I was pretty sure back ailments weren't treated with arts and crafts. "Okay," I promised her. "I'll do it."

For a kid with my neurological wiring, Show and Tell was pure hell, and I thought I was done for a while. I also knew the other kids would rather take a nap or eat library paste than listen to me talk about "sciatica." But my mother was adamant. The only way I could redeem the family honor was to once again face the fire by going back on the dreaded chair.

In the history of this time-honored school tradition, I may very well have delivered the first Show and Tell correction. "Uh, about what I said yesterday," I rambled on, acknowledging how I'd screwed up the details, hadn't gotten the facts straight. I talked about my dad's back problem, how he'd hurt it lifting some unknown object. I provided the name of a hospital my mother made me memorize, a name other than the one we visited. Just to be on the safe side, I mentioned the name of the actual hospital he was in and told them, "Be sure to tell your mom and dad that we *didn't* go to *that one*." I stressed the importance to my classmates of relaying this exact information to their parents that afternoon. Right away.

Looking back, this incident is where my biochemistry and environment merged into full-fledged neurosis; they were glued like tiles in an ashtray or stitched like a moccasin. It is when I began linking success with unnecessary guilt. If I feel good about it, there must be something wrong.

It is also, much later in life, where I began to recognize the absurdity of it all. I think about the seriousness with which I addressed my fellow five-year-olds, their minds most likely focused on when the milk cart would arrive. I think about the lesson my mother instilled, that lying is better than revealing mental illness. I ponder the real lesson, which is this: no one cares as much as we think they do.

Despite disguising my own mental illness over the years, the rants I've spewed about how society doesn't "get it," and the reality that mental health is often still taboo, I can still see decades of progress. My friends and I talk about our antidepressants the way others talk about blood pressure medication. There is no shame, only shared experience and gratitude for improved health.

When the clouds of shame are at their darkest, I wonder how much of the shadow is my own. Am I embarrassed because of what other people may think, or is the five-year-old inside of me still trying to hide the family secrets? Tolerance and understanding grow through openness, and I'm working to be more open. And, odds are, when we are feeling self-conscious, most people hearing our stories are like those kindergarteners waiting for the milk cart.

*Sherry Vondy Beaver is a project manager and writer, whose work ranges from jokes to academic journal articles. Currently she is co-writing a novel. She lives in Eugene, Oregon, where the air smells like blackberries.*

# ROCK BOTTOM
## Marcia Kester Doyle

*T*he well is deep, and beneath the murky water at the bottom lies the secret place where fear and sorrow hide. This is the place that haunts my
dreams, a world of seamless shadows tearing at the fabric I've carefully woven
to mask what sleeps inside me. Hopelessness, emptiness, deceptively calm waters drowning my soul as it slips beneath the depths of depression to rock bottom. Many people try to fix me, but no one can throw the rope that will pull
me out of the darkness.

My eyes are reflected in the water's smooth surface, the curve of the iris
where it meets the black onyx pupil. There, beneath the green blue shade so
similar to the sea, is sorrow. A defining moment that has shaped who I've become. Years of tangled emotions fall like bitter rain from my eyes and threaten
to pull me under. The bite of a blade against my pale wrist—sharp teeth that
draw the first beads of blood.

I was only sixteen years old when I first started cutting my wrists
and forearms with the sharp knives from my mother's kitchen
drawer.

Depression has shadowed me since childhood. I never felt comfortable in my own skin, but I was too young to understand what caused me to feel things more deeply than others. I only knew that I was different. I wept at the beauty of the setting sun at the end of each day because it felt like a small death inside me. No one ever said that it was unhealthy for a six-year-old to wake each morning with a sense of dread, because they never had the chance. I was too ashamed to tell anyone how I felt.

My grade school years were a mixed bag of insecurities that compounded the depression issues. I ran home from school often, cutting through neighborhood yards to escape the children who taunted me. I was a shy, pudgy little girl who struggled in school and dealt with an eye condition known as mixed dominance, requiring me to wear a patch over one eye. This made me an easy target for the bullies who thrived on breaking me down in order to build themselves up. The insecurities created from this situation festered deep inside me, feeding my depression and causing years of fear and shame during my time in grade school. My parents, sensing something was wrong but unable to get me to discuss my feelings, sent me to a therapist. I resented the intrusive questions he used in an attempt to chip away at the walls I'd carefully built. Being sent to his office once a week reinforced what I knew all along—I was broken and unfixable.

Since there was a negative stigma attached to depression during those days, I learned to mask what I considered my abnormality with humor. But it went beyond hiding what was tearing me up inside. The shame I felt was carefully concealed under the long-sleeved shirts I wore to cover the self-inflicted wounds on my arms. Cutting myself was the coping mechanism of choice for the unexplainable, inner turmoil that plagued my life. It became a cleansing ritual of sorts— the blood a punishment for the ugliness I felt inside.

It wasn't until I enrolled in a fine arts school that I discovered there were others like me—people who expressed their raw emotions through art. I worked out my demons through writing while they painted, danced, created music, and immersed themselves in dramatic roles on stage to combat the depression that haunted them.

I thought I'd finally escaped the sadness that had once consumed me. It was always there on the fringes of my life, but I was able to skirt the depression by keeping busy with my studies and surrounding myself with supportive friends. The emotional boost I received from writing gave me the confidence I needed to keep the sadness and anxiety away. For the first time, I experienced real happiness.

I felt happy, that is, until I fell in love with the wrong man. He was charming, handsome, and supportive of my goals. Within a few months we moved in together, and I thought I was living a fairy tale. People tried to warn me; they saw a darkness in him that I was too blind to see. He loved me, and that was all that mattered.

It didn't take long before his true colors emerged in the form of alcohol and drug abuse, but I naively believed that I could fix him. I thought if I loved him harder, he would change. But the more he drank, the meaner he became. Over time, he chipped away at my confidence by berating me, hitting me, locking me in rooms for hours on end and threatening my life. After one particularly heated argument, he hit me so forcefully that I fell backwards onto the hard asphalt and shattered my elbow. Although a small voice inside me knew that I had become a victim of his sick cycle of physical abuse, I allowed it because I'd fallen into the sinkhole of his lies that I was worthless and unlovable. The murky waters of depression washed over me once again, dragging me down to the rocky depths below.

I stayed in the abusive relationship for over a year, numb to his words and the fists that no longer hurt. I thought of suicide daily— death was preferable to feeling nothing at all. I was living in a muted world, trapped underwater in an emotionless sea. I stood on the edge of the cliff, looked down into the dark void of nothingness and heard a small voice telling me to jump. I just wanted to be free.

Call it what you want, a higher power or intuition, but something stopped me from carrying out my plan to overdose on medication.

Within a few weeks, I met someone special who became a positive force in my life. He was a gentle man who had survived a difficult and painful childhood. As a young boy, he'd been adopted twice, experienced the death of his mother and was later left by the father who divorced his second adoptive mother. Despite the losses in his childhood, he was the happiest, most dependable person I'd ever met. He embraced life to the fullest and sought the positive side in every situation he encountered. It was his unconditional love that pulled me out of the dark well of depression and into the light.

We've been married for thirty years now, that gentle man and I, and for the most part, they have been years of joy. As with any marriage, our wedding vows came with the emotional baggage of our pasts. We've been through family deaths, marital problems, job losses, financial woes, teen problems, and health issues. But I am fortunate enough to have a husband who views my depression in an objective manner, accepting the fact it is a chemical imbalance over which I have no control. Although he often feels helpless when my depression strikes, he is supportive and rides out the storms with me when I feel overwhelmed. This has meant filling the shoes of both mother and father during the days when I would cry uncontrollably and lacked the energy or motivation to get out of bed.

In the early years of our marriage, I kept track of my bouts of depression to understand what was triggering it, disregarding the moments of ordinary sadness associated with stressful life events. I focused instead on the root of the despair that occurred for unexplainable reasons, and I discovered a definite correlation between the fluctuating hormones of my menstrual cycle and my depression. Even so, I was still concerned people would view me as weak and unstable. I wrote off my symptoms as general PMS—something I could learn to control on my own, rather than seeking professional advice.

It took years of battling the escalating depression in my late forties before I realized I needed help waging the war against losing my sanity. The onset of menopause only intensified the depressive symptoms I felt, stranding me in a bleak landscape of hopelessness. My rapid mood swings were affecting the stability of my family and wreaking havoc on my life. I had to accept I had a disease, and it needed to be treated by a medical professional. Thankfully, with the encouragement of family and friends, I was able to put fear and guilt aside to find a treatment that worked for me. My doctor prescribed an antidepressant, and it has made a world of difference in the quality of my life.

There are still days that are rougher than others, but the medication keeps the feelings of utter hopelessness and despair at bay. I am able to handle stressful situations more easily and have found that along with medication, humor and writing are my best coping mechanisms. The compassion and understanding I've received from my family gives me hope and the courage to change.

*The well is deep, yet in its darkness, there is light. The sun glistens like a thousand stars on the water's surface, chasing shadows that once clouded the sky. Listening closely, I hear the voice that heals the broken soul. There is so much more to live for.*

*Marcia Kester Doyle is a native Floridian and a married mother of four children and has one feisty grandchild. She is the author of the humorous blog,* Menopausal Mother, *where she muses on the good, the bad and the ugly side of menopausal mayhem. She is a contributing writer for* Huffington Post, In The Powder Room, What The Flicka *and* Humor Outcasts. *Her work has also appeared on* Scary Mommy, Blunt moms, BlogHer, Lost In Suburbia, The Erma Bombeck Writers Workshop, Midlife Boulevard, BA50 *and* The Woven Tale Press *among others. She is the author of the humorous book,* Who Stole My Spandex? Midlife Musings From A Middle-Aged MILF *and is also an author/contributor to six other books. Marcia is a* BlogHer Voice Of The Year 2014 *recipient and her blog* Menopausal Mother *won* Voice Boks Top Hilarious Parent Blogger 2014. *She was also voted top 25 in the* Circle Of Moms *contest 2013.*

# ON THE STREETS

## Brad Shreve

F lat broke and rent past due I was days away from being on the streets. For the first time in my thirty-five years of working, I was fired from a job. The racing thoughts and distraction of mania made it nearly impossible to focus on the intricacies of my job in computer programming. I had been warned several times that I needed to be more productive, and I tried. I had never worked faster or harder, but I continued to fail. My inability to focus resulted in many projects started, but few finished.

I had no idea my efforts were being hampered by mania. I had not yet been diagnosed with bipolar disorder. My employers gave me a generous severance package but, unfortunately, I was on a manic high when I was fired. Typical for me, the money was spent quickly and frivolously. Within a week, my only financial buffer to protect me while I searched for a new job was gone.

I thought I was prepared for the worst until I met Scott at a bar at closing time. Knowing my predicament, he offered to let me stay on his couch, but I quickly learned that his generosity came at a heavy price. Scott expected sex in return for providing a roof over my head. I believed I had no other option than to oblige.

My child support payment was coming up and I had no idea how I was going to pay it. Of all the money I owed, this was the one thing I refused to accept I could not pay. Fortunately, because I'm a recovering alcoholic, which is considered a disability, I qualified for emergency income through Social Security. Just in time, my first $600 was deposited into my account. My child support payments were $500. I took the money from my account and made plans to get a money order the next day.

The following morning there was a monsoon where I lived in southern California. The deluge of runoff water turned the streets into raging rivers. I put my wallet in my back pocket and headed out the door for the money order. Three blocks away, as I neared the bus stop, I reached back to get my bus pass, but my wallet was gone. Did I forget it? I knew I hadn't. I then discovered I was wearing my jeans with the hole in the back pocket. Only, it was no longer a hole—there was no longer a bottom to the pocket at all and I realized my wallet must have slipped out and likely would be back in my bedroom. As I ran back to the house, I watched the gushing water flow down the street and pour into the sewer grates. Knots were forming in my stomach and I prayed my wallet was still in the house. It wasn't.

Angry and scared, I gathered some hope and went back into the torrential rain to try and find the wallet. I retraced my steps up the hill to the bus stop, but the wallet was nowhere. I retraced my steps back down the hill, but still could not find it. Reaching my breaking point, I stood in the middle of the street in utter disbelief, my anger turned into despair as the pouring rain beat down even harder. Cold and soaked, I looked around. The only dry spot I could see was a small patch at the door to the church I was standing in front of. I walked up the steps to the door, put my back against it and slid down to the concrete below. I wanted to scream at the world, scream at God, but I didn't. Instead I put my arms around my knees, bowed my head and cried. I pictured what I must look like to all those passing by and all I could think was, "How pathetic."

In the days and weeks that followed, I continued to think about how pathetic my life had become. Although I was not yet diagnosed with bipolar disorder, I had been diagnosed with depression when I was fourteen and I could feel it coming. I decided I could no longer sell my soul for a place to live. With great fear of the unknown, I packed my duffle bag and left with no idea where I would live. I never saw Scott again.

Now homeless, each morning began with me having to find a place to hide my duffle bag. It contained all my belongings, but was too heavy to carry throughout the day. Besides, the last thing I wanted was to appear homeless. I didn't want to look like *those* people. After hiding my bag, I had to find food, turn in job applications, and because I had nowhere to go, I usually attended three Alcoholics Anonymous meetings a day. This much I accomplished on my good days.

Many days my depression was too strong to fight. I didn't want to kill myself—that would require too much effort. I just wanted to curl up and die quietly. On these days, I had to find a place for myself as well as my bag. Usually, I was hidden between shrubberies on the grounds of city hall. I would toss my bag on the ground, curl up next to it and use it as a pillow. I'd cry until I was too exhausted to cry any more. Was my depression worse because of my situation or was my situation worse because of my depression? I never was sure where the horrible cycle began, I only knew I was trapped.

I struggled equally with the nights. The best nights were when I had spare change because I could use it for bus fare. I knew the longest bus routes in the city and used that knowledge to my advantage. It was the optimum way to get a long stretch of sleep until the bus reached the end of the line when all passengers were required to get off the bus for fifteen minutes. The driver took her break and turned the bus around. Then it was back on the bus for another stretch of sleep.

Additional fare was required to take the bus back to the other end. This meant I was frequently stuck because I'd run out of money, trapped in one of the seedier areas of downtown Los Angeles or in downtown Santa Monica. Being in downtown Los Angeles, near the area called Skid Row, was terrifying. I would have to find a doorway to curl up in and guard my duffle bag the entire night. Falling asleep was too dangerous. Sleeping provided too much of an opportunity to have my belongings stolen, and many of the other homeless around me were willing to cause physical harm to get my stuff. As long as I stayed awake I was able to protect myself, and my bag.

Downtown Santa Monica, on the opposite end of the line, was a much better place to be stranded. It was downright luxurious in comparison. City ordinances outlawed sleeping in doorways or parks, but benches were open season. I was never able to find an empty bench downtown, which left me with only one option: the Santa Monica Pier. Although the pier is a tourist attraction, I was surprisingly left alone by the police and security guards.

I always chose a bench under the Ferris wheel even though it was more exposed to the cold ocean breezes; it was a bit more isolated from the other benches, which allowed me some privacy. Looking outside myself, I could see my life and I was disgusted with how far I had fallen. I knew I needed help; the depression was killing me. In time my cycle changed to a state where I was more balanced. Temporarily safe between mania and depression, I was finally in a frame of mind to seek the help I needed. I went to the closest L.A. County mental health clinic and waited an entire afternoon to see a counselor. The day ended and I was turned away, and told to arrive earlier the next day. As instructed I went to the clinic at the time they opened the next day. Once again, when it was time to close, I was turned away and told to try again the next day.

Finally, on the third day at the clinic they called my number before closing. I spoke with the admissions clerk for approximately fifteen minutes before he excused himself and walked away into a back room. I didn't understand that he was not a doctor; I expected him to return with a prescription. After another fifteen minutes, the clerk returned with the news that they would not take me as a client because I was too high-functioning. *Too high-functioning? I was living on the streets, scavenging each day for something to eat, yet they considered me too high-functioning!* I asked if I could please speak with a doctor, but was refused.

The clerk then proceeded to say the saddest words I had ever heard: "When you get worse, come back and we'll see if we can assign you a doctor then." He did not say, "if you get worse," but, "when you get worse." I was in shock. I had no idea what to do. I didn't want to get worse. Homeless, jobless, and now refused medical care? Suicide started to look like my best option.

After a month of being homeless, I had a conversation with a man at an Alcoholics Anonymous meeting. I'd seen him around, but never said more than hello. After we talked for a few minutes, he excused himself, talked to some people I knew and had them take me to the emergency room. I had no idea the man was a psychiatrist nor do I recall what I said to him, but whatever I said clued him in that I was suicidal.

When I arrived at the emergency room, the admitting psychiatrist had me placed on a 72-hour lockdown suicide watch. On the third day, my stay was extended for seven more days. On day nine, the day before being released, a psychiatrist called me into his office and told me I'd likely be on antidepressants for the rest of my life. It was not a surprise. He wrote me a prescription and told me that I'd been assigned a doctor at one of the county mental health clinics.

The clinics in my immediate area were understaffed, so the only clinic where they were able to place me was a 3-hour bus ride each way. The long rides gave me too much time to think about how far I had fallen. I nearly gave up, but fortunately the medication made me more stable than I had been. I was able to secure a job as a telemarketer, which allowed me to pay my child support and secured me a bed in a sober living facility. My circumstances were not where I had envisioned myself at forty years old, but I finally had hope, and that was more than I'd had for a very long time.

*Brad Shreve was diagnosed with bipolar disorder at the age of 45 and began blogging almost immediately afterwards. His blog, originally named "How is Bradley," was awarded by Psych Central as one of the top ten bipolar blogs in 2008. He was recently featured on Dr. Sanjay Gupta's website, "Health Matters." Like many on psychiatric medication, Brad gained a significant amount of weight, topping off at 303 lbs. In addition to writing about life with bipolar disorder, he reluctantly records his weight loss struggle. Originally from North Carolina, Brad lives with his husband, Maurice, in the Los Angeles South Bay. He is a writer. He can be reached at* insightsbipolarbear.com.

# THE HILARITY OF OUR COURTSHIP

## Carin Ekre Anderson

My husband Jesse and I just celebrated our fifth anniversary. I think that's pretty awesome for two people who have realized that nothing goes as planned. Hell, coming from the girl who was diagnosed with bipolar at age 15, I never planned on having any kind of good life. Two hospitalizations and a laundry list of failed meds kind of dashes the whole *hope for the future* thing, but I got lucky and found my fairytale, sort of. We've had our share of ups and downs and both agree that The Man Upstairs has a fantastic sense of humor. After all, he took two small-town kids destined for marriage, and placed them ten miles apart for their entire childhood, but didn't let them meet until their mid-twenties. And even then, they didn't meet until both had officially sworn off love for good.

One of the first times my husband-to-be laid eyes on me I was jumping around on a bar top, red curls flying, stomping and dancing for all I was worth to Miranda Lambert's 'Kerosene'. "I'm givin' up on love 'cause love's given up on meeeee!" It's a good thing I can carry a tune. In his version of events he raises his eyebrows and says to his pal Doug, "Wow … that's crazy." To which Doug replies, "Maybe you'll find out." Thanks guys. *Really.* Turns out he *would* find out (in more ways than one).

We had mutual friends who saw an opportunity, and so began their covert setup. Over the next few weeks we went on several group outings, but we were both still clueless about everyone's master plan. One night we randomly bonded over a conversation about playing acoustic guitar, and I offered to teach him. As I walked out to my truck we arranged a time to get together. I hollered out a "Rock on!" and threw up my hand for a high five, and somehow it turned into our first kiss. To this day we have no idea who kissed whom.

Our next date was chopping and stacking logs at my little house in the woods. Being the starving artist type I had run out of propane, but was lucky to have a wood stove for backup. As I sat complaining I was too small to chop wood, Jesse smiled his megawatt grin and offered to help.

"Dude, you can't come cut wood for me."

"Why not?" he says, "I like cutting wood."

And so he did. When we finished, I offered to take him out for a beer as a thanks for his help. We walked in and ordered, and honestly the work of stacking logs had my legs feeling like wet noodles. I moved to cutely hop up onto a stool, and in my mind it goes like this: I smile adorably and he sees how lovely and dainty I am and decides he's just crazy about me. However, what actually happened is like something out of a terrible rom-com, maybe starring Anna Farris or someone equally annoying. My super-klutz self decided she must make herself known, so I tossed my ponytail as I leapt on legs as unsteady as a baby fawn's and over the other side of the stool I went. My arms and legs flailed in midair and I landed on my ass and smacked my head. Awesome. As an added bonus I noticed, as I sat on the floor, that I was sticky and sweaty and I smelled less than fabulous. Ugh. *What a damn fine impression I've made.* Jesse suppressed a chuckle and helped me up. He was a keeper, so I invited him to an outdoor party my band was playing at and silently swore to myself I would do more yoga so I could finally become balanced and graceful … or at the very least a little less ridiculous.

The night of the party I was dressed to the nines and ready to belt out some serious rock n' roll. I was super stoked to see his face in the crowd, and was glad I'd get a chance to show off in hopes of making a better impression on him. That is until I was literally caught with my pants down. I'd snuck away to pee ('cause that's just how we do in northern Minnesota) and Jesse unknowingly startled me mid-stream in the outdoor semi-private facilities of the bushes.

"Hey, I wanted to ask, uh … will you be my girl?"

I barked out an involuntary laugh and asked, "Do people even do that anymore?" I then gracefully fell back, toward my own pee puddle. In the nick of time he gallantly reached out and took a hold of my hand. I grabbed his hand and simultaneously hunched over to protect the view of my lady junk as I pulled up my pants. It was so very awkward. I felt like a total asshole for sticking my giant foot in my giant mouth but I replied, "Sure. I'd like that. Nothing too serious though." I think at that point the irony of us both wanting to avoid love yet rapidly falling into it was lost on us.

Eventually we did all the cutesy couple things, and one night we found ourselves parked and stargazing. I needed a better view so I rolled down my window and sat on the ledge of it while leaning my head back toward the sky. Somehow I lost my grip on the roof and instantly slid back. I dropped straight out of the window of his truck and landed on my back in the dirt with my feet in the air. I was pretty sure he must be wondering how, exactly, he came to be dating Minnesota's own version of Mary Catherine Gallagher. Not for the first time, nor the last, I heard him suppress his laughter.

"Holy crap! Are you okay?"

"Yup. I'm fine."

The pain was intense and I thought I had just broken my ass, but I was not about to admit it. While lying in the dirt, I was seriously considering giving up on our relationship. Every time we got together I ended up making myself look more and more ludicrous. As we drove back to my house I hatched a plan that would definitely redeem me.

When we arrived, I excused myself to go to the bathroom and dug out my sexiest black lingerie. I owned that shit, man. I strutted and swung my hips like I was on the catwalk in Milan, and I could tell by the look on his face that he appreciated it. I decided to up my game. A little hair toss and—*oh damn! Houston, we have a problem!* I'm still not sure exactly how it all went down, perhaps too many things swinging and swishing at once, but the end result was me in a pile with a twisted ankle. I don't know how a person manages a sprain with bare feet, but holy hell I did it. He rushed over to me and I yelled, "No! I don't need help!" while I hid behind my hair. I am a total dick when I get hurt, and this was Jesse's introduction to that fun little piece of me. I decided immediate escape was best, but I couldn't stand so I crawled all the way back to my bedroom to get dressed, thonged butt sticking up the whole way. When I came out we watched a movie and I pouted all night. I'm a real charmer.

After that I learned how to laugh at myself just a little bit, and we actually had some dates where I did not look like a human caricature of the Tasmanian Devil.

On Valentine's Day he told me to dress up, so I did. I didn't know where we would be going and it was a wonderful surprise when we pulled up in front of one of my favorite places. Ridiculous as usual, I salivated over the menu and talked too loudly while we waited for our table to be ready. As we sat I remarked on how nice it was that they decorated the tables with such lovely bouquets, but halfway through our meal I realized that only our table had such an arrangement.

"Hey! Are these for me?" Duh. Classy through and through. We were waiting for dessert when Jesse scooted his chair closer to mine and began talking about how much he adored me. *Swoon.* I wondered where all this came from, because he's definitely no wordsmith. This sounded incredibly well thought out. *Wait a minute … what's going on here?*

"Oh whatthefuck!" I blurted out with a wide grin.

"Um, yeah!" Jesse said, as he blushed seven shades of crimson. "I'm trying to ask you to marry me, sweetheart."

That's me, folks. The woman who said "fuck" at her own proposal *before* she said yes. What can I say? He caught me by surprise.

Hard to believe, but I grow more awkward and clumsy by the day. I am lucky enough to have married someone who enjoys laughing with … er, *at* me. A man who knows that some of my shenanigans come from the manic side of my illness, and understands that some of my darkness is from the flip side of that coin, and will never let me be silly or sad alone. I'd have never thought that such ridiculous things could lead to a happy ending for a girl who was once so broken.

*Carin Anderson is a married to the love of her life, Jesse, and is the mom to her wonderful four year old son Leonidus. She was diagnosed with Bipolar Disorder at the age of 15. She spent the next ten years searching for the right medical team who has now helped her live her life on a balanced path with the right coping skills and medication. With the support of her big loud amazing family she has found peace in life and enjoys her many hobbies of being a musician, singer, songwriter, and a writer. She is most happy to just be herself.*

# AN UNFORGETTABLE SCAR

## Andrea Keeney

A meeting room is simply a vacant area, until it is filled with a group of people who have something in common. Something that bonds each individual as a cohesive unit. For me and seven other individuals, that bond was suicide. We had all tried it. We had all failed. Therefore, we were all sentenced to intensive outpatient therapy in the hopes that a good dose of counseling and some heavy duty antidepressants would keep us from trying to kill ourselves again.

We were women of varying ages; some of us were wives, some widows, and some of us mothers. We were all different, but we each had a unifying scar. Some carried their scars on the walls of their stomachs from the bottles of pills they swallowed. Others, such as myself, carried our scars as visible marks along the deep blue veins that stretched the length of our wrists. We held our wounds tight to us, hiding them under sleeves, covering them with bandages and bracelets. We kept them to ourselves, holding the darkness close to our hearts.

I kept my scar smothered below bandages and a thick layer of clothes. I refused to speak of it and refused to share with the seven other women around me. I held my scar tightly in part because of fear that they wouldn't understand what drove me to try to end my life. They wouldn't understand the obsessions that played endlessly in my mind, spinning like a carousel that never stopped. They wouldn't understand my illness: obsessive-compulsive disorder. It's a misunderstood disease, usually thought of as a few obsessions or a few small fears, like a fear of germs. It means being extra neat and tidy, right? Most people don't know about the intrusive thoughts. They aren't aware of the kind of obsessions I dealt with. The darker obsessions, like my fear of accidentally hurting my child and my fear of being a bad mother, of being such a bad person that my life is not worth living. Most people overlook the crippling anxiety because they can't see the rapid heartbeat and racing pulse, or the moments of terror and unrelenting, unstoppable thoughts.

I hid my scar out of fear, but also out of guilt. Guilt over a disease I couldn't control. Guilt for all the ways I'd fallen short of the mother I wanted to be, which I felt in very small ways as I looked at my children. It was like an extra tug in the pit of my stomach that never really went away. It was there because I would always remember that at one time I was not there for my children. At one time I was not strong. For every ounce of guilt that I felt there came a small amount of uncertainty. Would the disorder take me from them again? Would the anxiety cripple me? Would the intrusive thoughts change me, and in turn change the mother I thought I would be?

I held my guilt just as closely to my heart as I held my scars. I shouldered it alone. My therapist knew that. I suppose that's why he called on me that day. That's why he placed his pen and paper on the wood table and quietly said my name.

"Andrea. I don't think we've heard from you yet."

I pulled my sleeve further down over my wrist and crossed my arms over my chest. My hands started to sweat and my mouth went dry. My heart began to race, but the anxious thoughts seemed distant—an attractive side effect of the large doses of antipsychotics I'd been ordered to take. All seven women turned toward me. Most of them smiled encouragingly, though their enthusiasm didn't help.

Finally, I gulped hard and cleared my throat. "I didn't plan it," I mumbled. "The suicide. It just ... happened." I sighed, looked down at my bandaged wrist, and recalled how I found myself terrified to step out of my shower. How the heavy drops of water did nothing to slow the way my mind was flooded with thoughts of what a terrible person and mother I was. How I strained to breathe through the anxiety and how every single inch of me wanted nothing more than to sit with my family. I wanted nothing but to stand in the presence of my husband and two daughters without fighting back my fears of being near them. Of accidentally hurting them. Of being unworthy to breathe the same air as them.

But try as I may the thoughts didn't stop. They didn't slow. Not even as I let the water fall around me. Not even as I stood motionless, listening to the drops of water along the shower floor. When the obsessions would not stop I looked for refuge, for a way out. For a way to keep my children and my husband from being hurt, from being near me. Refuge came in the form of a razor. It sat directly in front of me, in the same place it had been for the past week, though I didn't notice it until that moment. But once I saw it, once I found the thing that would free my family from me, I didn't waste a moment. I held it tight in my hand and pressed the blades against my wrist.

It barely broke my skin.

I tried again, pressing the blade harder against my wet skin. The sting of the metal pulling at my flesh brought tears to my eyes. A few drops of blood pooled around the cut. I thrust my arm under the warm water, watching as the red liquid streamed down my arm. The cut wasn't deep enough. I knew I hadn't nicked the vein, so I tried again and again. And again. Over and over I pulled the razor down my arm; each time I pressed harder. With each slice the sting dulled until it all but vanished. Until my skin was swollen and red. Until the warm water rushed along my cuts and carried my blood away. Until my hand slipped.

The razor fell to the shower floor. It clanged against the hard surface, sending echoes through the small, steam-filled room. For a moment I watched as blood swirled around the razor. I looked to my wrist. I hadn't hit the vein. There wasn't enough blood. Tears streamed down my cheeks and my knees grew weak. I took a seat on the shower floor. I couldn't move, couldn't stand the thought of leaving the shower, of facing my family. I let the water run over me until it grew cold. Until goose bumps formed on my skin and I started to shiver. Just minutes out of the shower, my husband saw the cuts. He called the doctor, found a family member to watch the girls, and before I knew what was happening he drove me the doctor's office.

"And that's why I'm here," I finished.

I didn't look up. I ended the session in silence. I never spoke of the suicide attempt again, but I never forgot it. Even now, nearly four years later, I cannot forget it. Just as I cannot forget the illness that lives within me. The illness that I carry, that I am forced to survive. I cannot forget it, and so I carry it. I live with guilt and uncertainty and a question that I am unable to answer: How is it possible to not hate yourself, when such a large part of who you are is an illness you detest? I wonder if I will ever answer this question. Perhaps I cannot answer it. I must simply live with it.

*Andrea Keeney is a chef, driver, booger-wiper, master of dance parties, laundry expert, and CEO of family affairs. In short, she is a mother and wife. When she isn't navigating the rough terrain of parenting, she is writing. Andrea is the author of the hilarious book,* Moms: As Elite as the CIA...Well Almost, *as well as the creator of the blog* Parenting with Parents.

# THE REAL HUNGER GAMES

## Carrie Groves

I have always been very aware of my weight. I can remember standing on the scale when I was a young girl, horrified that I crossed the threshold of sixty pounds. I don't know how old I was, but if the weight of my children is any indication, I couldn't have been more than eight.

Eight years old.

Way too young to be worried about how much I weighed. I should have been thinking about what the Snorks were going to do on their next adventure or if Jem would ever be rid of the Misfits. Instead, I worried about my appearance. In my reality, the size of my waist was inversely related to the size of my self-esteem.

Due to my internal struggles with my weight, I have always been hyper-aware of the dieting and eating habits of the people around me. As they applauded themselves for losing weight or beat themselves up for gaining a few pounds, I learned that being thin meant being happy. I often heard, "You can never be too rich or too thin."

Taking it to heart, I became a child obsessed. I remember sitting down and noticing my thighs had spread out. I grabbed ahold of a chunk of "fat" and showed it to my friend saying, "Look at this! It is so disgusting!" I was twelve years old and fixated on my size, viewing everything in extremes.

The formative years were difficult for me. I was bullied for being smart, for my bad perm, my glasses, and my all-around dorkiness. I tried so hard to fit in with the most popular girls in my middle school, but was only able to crack the outer walls of their sanctified group. I later learned they didn't even like each other that much. I was living the 1992 version of Mean Girls. Their cruelty did little to curb my appetite for being included in their pack. I jumped up and down trying to get them to accept me, but they never did. I always felt so very alone.

The summer between middle school and high school I blossomed from an ugly duckling into a beautiful swan. My hair grew out of its frizzy, Toni home perm. I got contact lenses and discovered the magic of makeup. I thought all my problems had been solved; the friendships and camaraderie I had longed for would come now that I was pretty. However, my new beauty brought more trauma to my psyche instead of giving me the happiness I sought. I didn't know how to handle all of the attention, especially when it came to boys. For so long, I craved having people love me; I didn't know how to handle it when they finally did.

When boys talked to me, I felt anxious and tongue-tied. All I could think was, "Is my hair okay? Did I wipe my lunch off of my face? What if I have something in my teeth?" If I was lucky enough to know I was going to be talking to a member of the opposite sex, I would make sure I had plenty of talking points on hand, terrified that I would run out of things to say. I'm pretty sure I looked like a deer caught in the headlights. Between my expression, the sweat that exploded from my armpits, and the knot of anxiety that gripped my stomach, it's a wonder I talked to anyone at all.

The stress bottomed out what was left of my self-esteem. I had to look perfect all the time. I started binging and then drastically reducing my caloric intake as a way to balance my weight. I would eat a full dinner of my mom's amazing cooking before going out with friends and then I would eat chocolate cake with a side of French fries. The days were filled with endless cups of coffee. And when the pendulum swung too far in one direction, I would cut way back on my food intake and chew gum to stave off hunger pains.

In college, hiding became my specialty. I wore clothes that covered my midsection and hips, horrified at the thought of anyone seeing how disgusting they were. I layered on makeup to cover my imagined faults: dark circles, acne, visible pores, and laugh lines. During my freshman year, I became obsessed with working out. I started taking a cardio class, lifting weights, and trying to strengthen my bloated and distended core.

It didn't take long before I discovered purging. I was aware enough to know that throwing up and taking laxatives would damage my system, but I rationalized that ingesting natural laxatives, like raisins, was completely acceptable. I ate more raisins than one human being should eat in a lifetime. I also drank excessive amounts of coffee, avoided cheese, bananas and anything else that might negate the positive effects of my natural colon stimulants.

Between runs across campus, to the loo, and working out in my apartment, I was surrounded by a cloud of depression. All I did was think about food. Every morning I woke up starving. I immediately thought about what I would eat for lunch and how that would impact what I had for dinner. If I had something toxic, like carbohydrates, I would balance it out with steamed vegetables. There was a constant calculation of calories in and calories out. I was also plagued with the constant thought that I needed to exercise and run off whatever else I could to make my daily caloric intake negative.

I tried to combat what was going on in my head by research. If I understood what an eating disorder was, then I could control it, or at the very least use my knowledge to my advantage before the disorder paralyzed me. My research led me to the sad realization that, although I did suffer from an eating disorder, I had no desire to stop what I was doing. If I did that, then I would get fat, and I would have rather died than get fat. The thought of being obese horrified me. I felt like it was a slippery slope between neglecting my dietary maintenance or missing a workout and barreling to all-out fatness.

The rest of college I struggled with my hyper-awareness of my weight. I struggled with the constant balance of calories ingested against their inverse expended. I struggled with the need to work out regardless of what the scale told me. The entire time for me was marked with pain and sadness. Eventually I met a man who made me feel beautiful even when I was at my ugliest. For a few years, I was able to cope with what was swirling around in my head.

However, the birth of my first child, a son, threw me into my darkest period. This time the demon knocking at my door was not tied to my body image, but was postpartum depression. I was exhausted, teary, and detached from everyone around me. I chalked up my anguish to normal new parent emotions, but it lingered long after my son was sleeping through the night.

The hole I fell into was so dark and deep, it could have been Robert Frost's woods. And I had miles to go before I slept. Trudging along, I stopped eating, trying to find any way to stop my downward spiral. I felt like I was tumbling down a well, throwing my arms out to both sides, trying to slow down with no help in sight. There was nothing to grab onto to stop the free fall and so I just kept going further and further into the darkness.

One day I woke up and saw my weight had plummeted to 114 pounds. It was less than I weighed before I got pregnant. I knew I was unhealthy, but the only reason I focused on getting better was because I wanted to be there for my son. He was the bucket in the well that caught my fall.

Slowly I started to pull myself together. I stopped using the scale and counting calories. Every day I fought the voices in my head that told me I was fat and unlovable. I tried to push those thoughts to a small corner of my mind, and it was exhausting. I started taking antidepressants and tried to rebuild relationships with my friends and family. The battle was long and hard, but eventually I reached a tremulous place in the world by clawing my way out of the depth of my despair. I was fighting for my life so I could not only be a part of my son's life, but a positive role model for him.

Now, I also have a daughter who is intelligent, spirited, and spectacular. I do not want her to lose that delight and spark. I want her to be strong mentally and physically; I want her to love herself no matter what her body looks like. Every day I work to exhibit positive messages and try to show her what a healthy, strong woman looks like.

It's much easier said than done. I still struggle with negative self-talk and an overwhelming need to analyze every piece of food that enters my mouth. It has come to a point where I acknowledge that this demon is there, and I choose to ignore it.

One day I hope to talk to her about what I have been through and what I battle every day. I hope that it will empower her to become the woman she wants to be, unencumbered by her own psyche.

*Carrie Groves is the voice of Ponies and Martinis, a blog about her favorite things; kids, wine, and general life failures. When she's not writing, she is stumbling through life in the Midwest trying to raise two kids, three dogs, and one husband. Her work has been featured on BLUNTmoms and Mamapedia.*

# THE BIG SECRET
## Leigh Baker

Have you ever *pretended* to be drunk? No, I don't mean pretended to be sober; we've all miserably botched that. I mean pretend to be wasted when the strongest thing you've had is carbonated water. It's harder than you think.

I remember trying to appear inebriated at a Christmas party when I was pregnant with my second child. I'd had a few miscarriages after my first child and made the mistake of prematurely announcing each successive pregnancy, not anticipating any complications, much less losses. I decided to keep the expectant news to myself until I was assured and far enough along for people to wonder if I had eaten too many burritos or was, in fact, with child. I became pregnant with my son early in December and, although a merry gift indeed, it was a horrible time to be fake-drunk on the party circuit.

Nothing sends up red flags faster than a woman declining a little bubbly at a Christmas party, especially when I am the woman. In order to avoid the probing questions and curious glares, I devised a plan to get fake-drunk off a bottle of non-alcoholic red wine I cleverly hid under my bathroom sink.

*Cheers!* Merry Christmas! *Tink!* You look fabulous! *Tink! Tink!* I stealthily snuck off to refill my glass after each celebratory toast and acted progressively more belligerent as the night went on. I stumbled around my kitchen like a baby deer looking for its footing and laughed louder than anyone at my own jokes. My husband suggested I "tone it down" as I ascended the dining room table for all to see my Roger Rabbit. I was told I frequently behaved that way drunk, therefore I assumed people expected the same shenanigans of me that night as well. It wasn't easy, but I pulled it off and no one was wiser I was with child.

Pretending to be shit-faced is almost as hard as feigning happiness when you suffer from depression and anxiety. Depression has a way of robbing you of your senses, making somewhat simple tasks seem insurmountable. Forced slurred words and garbled laughter are met with the same strained worry as pushing a smile upwards or obliging unexpected phone calls or visitors—you're incoherent just the same. Despite everything, no one wants to be detected as a fake, a fraud, a counterfeit. Much like my stellar holiday-hammered performance, I've approached many parenting moments faking it. I overact, over-explain, and overindulge my children to hide any maternal insecurities I harbor from living with depression.

I remember when I faked my way through the dreaded sex talk with my daughter. I was too honest that day in an effort to conceal my underlying feelings of anxiety and perceived worthlessness as a mother. I feared that during these big moments—periods, boyfriends, and the sex talk—I would flub it up and she'd finally see me as the miserable imposter I was. Instead I am pretty sure I scared her for life, and myself too.

⟫ ⟪

My daughter was barely eight years old when she cooked up a minor illness, causing her to skip school for a day. Not just any day, but the day I had my annual OBGYN appointment. I had no option but to take her to the appointment with me. She had long outgrown the days when I could park her in the stroller facing the wall while my eyes locked and loaded on the tropical poster-covered ceiling tiles of the examination room.

I figured if she was old enough for lies, then she was old enough for truths. Being the over-explaining hipster I am I took her to Starbucks, got her a hot cocoa, and described precisely what she was going to see in the appointment. I delicately explained I would casually undress, lay on a papered table with my legs spread *very* far apart while a male doctor poked around inside my vagina, probably my anus too, and then feel all over my breasts just to make sure everything was working the way nature intended. After my 30-minute illustration, complete with a napkin schematic, I asked her if she had any questions. She reluctantly replied, "No."

The appointment went exactly as I had counseled and she behaved angelically. As soon as we got in the car I asked her if she had any questions about the appointment. She looked at me adorably and hit me with the one burning question I had not prepared her for.

"Mommy, remember when you told the doctor that you and daddy weren't going to have any more babies?" she said.

"Yes," I remembered.

"Well, how do you *not* have a baby?"

"Well, you just don't try to have a baby," I said as if that were enough.

"But how do you *not* have a baby?" She wasn't satisfied.

Obviously, that question requires knowing *how* to have a baby in order to understand how *not* to have a baby. Interesting—I didn't think this was how the big question was going to be posed and I needed a little more time to prepare my elaborate response and visual props.

"I'm glad you asked. I have a very informative book about this at home and I would love to read it with you tonight," I said.

That was enough to tide her over until bedtime.

She was bright-eyed and attentive as we snuggled into bed with the book *What's the Big Secret?* Before we got to the actual secret, we spent a few moments studying the anatomically correct graphics and discussing the differences between boys' and girls' bodies. I should explain that I've never been one to skip the entire region between the belly button and kneecaps, nor have I embraced pet names for body parts. It's a vagina; call it a vagina. Still, she was rather surprised to learn there were, in fact, three holes *down there.* The urethra, vagina and anus were the costars of our tale with sperm being the head-liner. After nearly thirty minutes, we were only on page three and still hadn't gotten to the *secret.* I had to move this expose along if she was going to get to sleep before midnight. Once we got to the actual secret, the book displayed a male graphic on the left side of the page and female graphic on the right side of the page. I carefully explained semen flowed out of the male through the penis (on the left page) and entered the vagina travelling upward to the ovaries (on the right page).

"Wait a minute," my daughter interrupted. "How does the sperm get from that page," she pointed to the left side of the book, "to that page?" She then hit the right page with her index finger.

I didn't want my innate fear and angst to take hold. Nevertheless, I felt myself wanting to say, *You just close the book! Voila! The pages touch!* But even in my despair I knew that wasn't the right thing to say, so I fake-drunk my way through the conversation. I explained that the penis actually had to go *inside* the vagina.

The big secret was revealed and boy (or girl), did she have questions. Her first inquiry was the most loveable.

"Mom, how much does it cost to adopt a baby?" she demanded to know.

Looking in her innocent blue eyes I said, "I don't know, honey, but Daddy and I will pay for it if you don't ever want to have sex." Perhaps it wasn't the best response but it was all I could think of in the moment.

This is where it got tricky.

"So only one sperm fertilizes the egg?" she confirmed over and over and over again, wondering if my answer would change. *Yes, only one sperm.* Being the natural Good Samaritan she is, she became frantic over the fate of the millions of other unsuccessful, less heroic sperm.

"Where do all the other sperm go?" she fretted.

"Well, they just go away," I stated, trying to avoid the word *die.*

"Where? Where do they go?" she wanted to know.

"They just come out."

"How?" she wondered.

"They just drip out," I said.

"Drip out where?" she said, unable to fathom what I was saying. "*Where* are they coming out?" She needed specifics.

"The same place they went in," I conceded.

"They drip out of your hole? Which hole? Why?" she bombarded me.

*OMG! Yes! They all drip out of your vagina hole! All the stupid, slow sperm drip out of your vagina onto your nice sheets for about twenty minutes unless you wobble to the bathroom and wipe your taint with a giant wad of toilet paper sending all the dumb, little motherfuckers down the drain. It's disgusting.*

"What happens after they drip out? Are they dead? Are they sad?" she persisted.

She focused on the three holes and dead ejaculate for nearly two hours while I faked my way through the logistics and possible emotions of sperm. My husband, who had known this bedtime discussion was taking place, finally approached the closed door, lightly knocked and posed the question, "Everything all right in here?"

I waved him in, exasperated by the adolescent interrogation. She looked up at him lovingly and said, "Daddy, can I ask you one question about the big secret?"

"Sure, sweetie," he said.

"Does sperm come out of your butt when you fart?"

"No! No! Never!" he exclaimed. He looked at me, "What the fuck are you teaching her?"

"The facts," I defended.

"Mommy, does sperm come out of *your* butt when *you* fart?" she turned to me.

"Not usually," I said by mistake. "I mean, not anymore," I corrected myself.

*There was that one time in college we tried it, but no, sperm doesn't usually come out of my butt when I fart,* I wanted to clarify.

Unlike the Christmas party, I had a real hangover from pretending to be something I wasn't—a relaxed, composed, self-assured mother. Besides, if I'm going to have any success as a mother living with anxiety and depression, I'm going to have to fake it 'til I make it. Let's be honest; in a world built on perception, isn't it more important that others believe me even if I don't believe myself?

*Leigh Baker's debut humorous memoir* Is My Crazy Showing? *will be released in Spring 2015. She is the outrageous personality behind reluctant-marathoner Steady Betty and writes at the utterly addictive blog Leigh Bones where exaggeration is her specialty. Leigh's philosophy is you can't hide crazy so you may as well embrace it. Leigh brings an honest, fresh and daring truth to the literary world. When she's not writing, she spends her time pestering the FBI for a job. Though she's a California girl at heart, she now lives in North Carolina with her husband, who she likens to Richard Gere in Pretty Woman, along with her two amazing children.*

# THE PASSWORD TO ANXIETY
## Kristin Kelley

I've been dealing with anxiety for the majority of my life. It has been coming and going in varying levels of intensity since I was nine years old. What always surprises me is how, over twenty years later, I still have never really grown accustomed to it. It mutates like a virus: same disease, but every time a little different, a little worse, always one step ahead. It is a brand new threat, and you're sure that *this one* is it.

After graduating college I was flying high. The world was my oyster, they told me. I was moving to a new city, living with good friends in a great apartment in a new metropolis, building the American dream on streets of sunshine gold and candy skies. During this bright period of transition, I never would have guessed the seeds of panic were incubating yet again

It took a little while for the optimism to fade, but it did, like the page of coloring book left in the backyard all summer long, until it is bleached and blanched and sad. Outside the reins of working toward a degree, life felt open and vastly empty. Time wiled itself away with nothing to mark it. The reality of the meaninglessness of life was coming closer; I was watching the bell jar descend over me.

I began waking up scared. The feeling that I was going to die soon snaked its way into my brain and became all-consuming. I could never quite accept the idea that my anxiety was lying, that my fears were unfounded; the feeling alone was powerful enough to convince me that it "meant" something. Only a Higher Power could give insight like this. Anxiety knew All. Everything was terrifying, though nothing made sense.

One weekend my roommates invited me on a weekend trip to Chicago, but because of my crippling fear of death I obviously couldn't get on a plane, so I politely declined. Hours after they left, I tried to prepare myself to spend the night alone for the first time in my life. Daylight was fading, casting long, yellow light and shadows across the apartment through the blinds. I went through my brain and my phone, searching for anyone I could ask to come spend the night with me or let me spend the night with them, but summers in San Diego aren't a popular time for people to be sitting around with no plans. I shut all the windows and blinds and turned on all the lights in every room, even the closets, to keep the night out. I turned on the television, putting in a disc of *Friends* so that the frenzy of commercials wouldn't send me overboard. I could feel fear pressing in on the outside, so I did everything I could to distract myself from it. I started baking cakes and cleaning the apartment, scouring with force and hoping to tire myself out, but there was still a flame in my mind, burning with fear. I pretended not to notice, but it kept me jittery and on edge.

Around two in the morning, I went into my bedroom without turning off any lights. I got into bed and curled up as far into the corner of the wall as I could. I would think that I had fallen asleep, until I heard a noise echo through the empty apartment. Images of murderers and psychotics bombarded my mind, embellished by the night and sleeplessness. I tried to shut my eyes, but instead would jolt awake with my heart slamming against my chest so hard that I was shaking. I swore I heard someone trying to open the door. I was convinced I heard a window shatter. I would not be able to rest until I went to investigate, saying a prayer and saying goodbye to life every time. Over and over I fell into a light sleep wherein I felt mostly conscious, flying awake at every creak and settling of the building.

When the sun finally rose, I felt comfort. Day had come and the murderers would go back to their alleys. I finally allowed myself to fall into the deep sleep I had deprived myself of in the nighttime hours.

The harsh *ding* woke me. I gasped for breath, twitching with nerves and clutching at my fiercely beating heart. Where was I? What was going on? Why was I alone? Another *ding* startled me; I saw my phone light up on my nightstand. My bedroom came into view. The dim light in the room, the vast shadows around me, told me that it was late in afternoon again, the threat of another night already on its way. I reached for my phone with arms and hands that were shaking uncontrollably. Anxiety, it seems, is electric.

The text read, "Michael Jackson is dead."

That was all it took. It was the password that unlocked an anxiety attack, the likes of which I had never seen before. I never knew that such a random incident could trigger an episode of this magnitude.

*This is it. Today is my last day. I won't see another sunrise. Why had I taken so much of life for granted? I don't have a future, today is the day. In a week people will be at my funeral. How is life so fickle?*

I was scared and filled with anguish that I wasn't even going to be able to see my mother one last time. I was hyperventilating, I couldn't feel anything, I couldn't think of anything but death, of the end, of how that was it. Where was my mother? I didn't want to die alone, I needed someone to be with me and squeeze my hand and send me off to the unknown with a promise that they would follow. I didn't want to die, but I could look down on myself, nothing was real, I wasn't controlling my eyesight. None of this meant anything, this apartment was just an illusion. Would my sisters get married? I couldn't feel the world around me. This was what dying felt like. I didn't want to die, but wounded animals aren't reasonable while they are dying; like a wounded animal, the panic and fear controlled me. I paced back and forth, running from wall to wall, crying and screaming, "I don't want to die! Don't let me die! Mommy, I don't want to die!" Two hours later, my mother was at my apartment, taking her grown child, her twenty-three-year-old daughter, the flawed outcast of society, back to her childhood home.

*Kristin is a California native with roots in France and New York City. She received a bachelor's degree from the University of California, Santa Barbara, and studied creative writing at Columbia University. Life with an alcoholic father triggered much of her struggles from a young age, which persisted through adulthood. The beneficiary from Kristin's work will be* Al-Anon, *a support program for individuals whose lives have been affected by alcoholics, and has been a saving grace in Kristin's life.*

# THE DEPTH OF THE DARKNESS
## Lea Grover

When my postpartum depression began to consume me, I didn't tell my husband how thoroughly I knew depression. More than any emotion, it defined my life before I met him. I had shielded him from the details of its severity, and found myself loathing him for that ignorance.

I hadn't told him I began contemplating suicide at eight-and-a-half. That as a child I lay in bed, staring hopelessly at the ceiling, rationalizing that I would sleep if I were dead. I walked into the kitchen and took Mom's largest knife. I stood on a stool in the weird darkness, staring at the blade, wondering how it would feel to have the metal slice through my skin, into my heart.

I had told my husband that I suffered through depression as I entered my teen years. I wore black and wrote bleak, earnest poetry about the futility of existence. He didn't know how every movement of my pen across the paper was agony; each breath was a painful reminder I still had to live. He didn't know that as a tween my parents had taken me to several psychologists, who prescribed sleeping pills and antidepressants I never took, hoarding them in a secret box.

He didn't know I'd kept a knife in my pocket when I was fourteen, cutting shallow lines into my arm to keep my thoughts from straying too close to the edge of what was conceivable. He didn't know I used a razor blade to carve the scars still dimpling my arm, and each cut had brought the abyss closer. He didn't know what my parents hadn't known, that my paintings and late night walks and endless muraling and stacks of filled journals were a chronicle of depression that never got better, that never lightened, only accumulated like the other mountains of evidence of my misery and isolation, crushing me beneath them. He didn't ask what my parents never asked: "Are you really okay?"

My parents had bigger fish to fry. My older sister was pregnant, threatening to keep the baby to punish the man who impregnated her. My younger sister was a walking ball of rage and confusion. My grandmother died of colon cancer, leaving my ailing grandfather suddenly their charge. My father's company faltered in the dotcom bust. They didn't need to know I was planning to make my exit.

But my husband did know about New Year's Eve, 1999. How I'd gone to a party at a friend's request, and when she hadn't shown up I'd been a lone freshman in a house full of seniors. How a boy from school had raped me while his friends laughed nearby and I lacked the strength to speak the words trapped inside me: *Please, somebody help me. Somebody save me from this...*

Ten days later, I caught my reflection in the mirror. "You have pretty eyes," I said. I froze, staring at myself. I looked like a stranger.

I went up to my room and took the hidden pills. Then I crept through the house emptying medicine cabinets. I took every aspirin. In between mouthfuls of pills, I wrote letters. To my parents, my friends, for my sisters to open at special birthdays, graduations, weddings.

I waited until the world felt electric. Until my arms wouldn't quite do what I told them, and I reached for my desk drawer, where I'd hidden a pint of tequila. All I needed to do was drink it, and I would slip away. I'd be asleep before the cocktail could kill me.

But I couldn't stand. I couldn't reach it. Instead I slipped back to my knees, and collapsed onto the bed. I felt my heart racing, so fast I was sure it would burst. I felt my breath come in irregular gasps, and despite my fear I felt relief that finally it would be over, and all the pain and shame and confusion would never touch me again.

I stared at the underside of my top bunk, marveling that I could be so afraid of the strange pulsing of my blood in my veins, and still so grateful it would end. I turned my head, and my neck jerked spasmodically at the gesture. I looked at the collage on my wall, tens of thousands of eyes, cut from magazines and taped to the wall over hundreds of sleepless nights. I looked into one large blue eye, and the world darkened around me.

It felt as though I were flying, floating into it. A round, blue, curving tunnel, I almost believed that around the next bend I would find where I was going. My heart raced, stopped, and raced again, and suddenly my pace slowed.

I floated, staring ahead at the steel blue void, and I felt an emotion, raw and real, however subtle. Not regret, not remorse, just a suspicious apprehension of the unknown.

Then suddenly, I was rushing backwards. My whole body ached with the momentum, every muscle screamed at the pace, and I squinted my eyes against a blinding light.

The moment I noticed I was staring at the lamp on my ceiling, I also became aware that my whole body was seizing, jerking across the bed.

*So this is how it ends,* I thought, my body lurching painfully beyond my control. My head caught in the ladder to my top bunk, and my shoulders wrenched to the side. I fell forward, onto my arm, and began to vomit.

My heart beat irregularly, starting and stopping, racing and slowing down, and I began to cry. I realized I would survive if I kept puking, but I could not find strength in my limbs to roll onto my back and choke.

I lay, twitching and crying and retching in near silence, believing survival was worse than death.

Hours later, sunrise glinted off the massive puddle of vomit on my floor, soaking into my blue chenille rug. I couldn't sleep with my brain buzzing from amphetamines. I couldn't move, my muscles torpid from sedatives. My heart beat lazily, slowed by aspirin and melatonin, but kept beating by the ephedrine.

I cursed myself listlessly for my impatience to die. *If you'd only taken the pills you saved, you'd be dead by now. Sedatives alone would have done it.*

After an hour, I heard my father's voice. "Lea! It's time to get up! You're going to be late for school!"

Apathy kept my eyes open. Half an hour passed, and he pushed open the door. For the first time since becoming aware that I would have to continue living, another human being spoke to me.

"God dammit, Lea! Couldn't you at least have tried to get to the bathroom?" He stormed out of the room again, and I felt tears trickle down my cheek. I still couldn't move my head, and as I finally drifted to sleep I wished never to wake up. I wished to be crushed under the weight of my depression, to simply will myself to be no more.

It was the weight I carried into my adulthood, my depression was my secret, tiny though I believed it might be. And while I learned to live through it, learned to treat it like a shadow in the back of my mind rather than a ravenous animal, I never escaped it entirely.

It followed me until I fell in love and got married and had children, and as night after night I slept natural sleep and dreamed happy dreams, I believed it was gone. But with the birth of my third daughter, it returned at full force.

I started dancing every morning with my children, hoping that might be some sort of cure. *Maybe the endorphins or some weight loss or just dance parties with my kids will knock me out of this funk.* I made videos of our dance parties and set them to music. The girls loved them so I threw my energy into spinning in endless circles with my daughters.

I jumped and kicked, twirled them around, lifted them into the air. They laughed and danced, and I put on a brave face and smile for them. I smiled for the camera set on the mantle, filming my children's happy childhood with their happy mother.

I went through the moves of spinning with my daughters, my heart heavy with constant, nagging weight. Out of nowhere I felt my face contort, I collapsed on the armchair and cried.

"What's wrong, Mommy?"

"I just need a hug, sweetie."

She wrapped her tiny arms around me, and I squeezed my eyes as tightly as I could, but the hollow in my chest grew. Another daughter bounced up and put her hand on my knee.

"Keep dancing, Mommy!"

But I couldn't. I glanced at the camera, and knew it was recording me.

"Why are you sad, Mommy?"

I held my breath, trying and failing to keep my voice even. "I'm not sad … I'm just tired."

"Why are you tired, Mommy?"

All I could do was stare at the three tiny faces I'd brought into the world, and try to imagine what it would be like to feel absolutely nothing about them. To not feel guilty and miserable and overwhelmed.

I looked at them and wished I didn't love them so much. It was too much to bear, this feeling.

"Why are you crying, Mommy?"

"I'm not crying," I gasped, tears pouring down my face.

"Please don't cry, Mommy."

The kids went to bed early and I sat in the living room, staring at the blackened television screen, wondering if running away would make me feel less trapped and alone. Thinking about leaving my house with its endless stacks of laundry and crumbs under the table. Leaving three flights of stairs that isolated me from even a trip to the grocery store.

A terrifying lightness filled my chest as I thought about abandoning my family, the people who touched me and kissed me and offered love, it physically pained me to feel. Without them, there would be nothing. Without them, I could get in the car, I could go straight into the water and let it swallow me.

I turned on my camera and watched the video. I watched my children's oblivious optimism, and saw in my face the same look I'd seen fourteen years earlier when I passed by a mirror and spoke to myself aloud.

Watching the video over and over, I heard myself whispering into the emptiness of the room.

*Please, somebody help me. Somebody save me from this…*

*Lea Grover is a writer and toddler-wrangler, living in Chicago. She waxes philosophic about raising interfaith children, marriage after cancer, and vegetarian cooking. Her blog,* Becoming SuperMommy, *won second runner up in Blogger Idol, and her work has been featured in the* Huffington Post, Alternet, *and her daughters' toy refrigerator door. Her writing can be found in the books,* My Other Ex: Women's True Stories of Leaving and Losing Friends, Motherhood May Cause Drowsiness, Listen To Your Mother: What She Said Then, What We're Saying Now, *and* The #NoMoreShame Project Anthology. *When she isn't revising her upcoming memoir, she can be found singing opera to her children or smeared to the elbow in Townsend pastels.*

# PILL-POPPERS' PARADE: ON THE ROAD TO 'SANITY'

## Lauren Stevens

Successive miscarriages triggered the daily panic attacks that rendered my chest so tight it could crack a nut. When my mind became completely cluttered and my thoughts riddled with self-sabotage, I finally sought professional help. I mean, it's not "normal" to be afraid to leave the confines of your own home, or to believe you'll be broadsided by a train each time you drive over tracks, is it? Getting effective mental health care was truly an obstacle course, as I jumped through the hoops of insurance companies and proved my craziness to medical professionals. It was a tumultuous time riddled with deception, temper tantrums (thrown by both my toddler and myself), and desperation.

Before receiving help, I had two discernible moods: Deeply Sad and Raging Anger. When I wasn't a motionless, weeping lump on the couch, I was an angry version of Tigger from Winnie the Pooh, ready to pounce, taking out my intense anger on anyone who dared cross my path. Telemarketers and slow checkout clerks were either conspiring against me or baiting me, so I snapped at them at the slightest sign of any snafu or unhelpfulness. I was actually hung up on by the billing rep at the hospital where my post-miscarriage medical procedures were performed, who mistakenly called me three times in one day after the billing manager had promised me they would stop calling. My wrath was so out of control that lashing out at a hospital system that had "mistreated me" with "harassing phone calls" made sense at the time. I look back with embarrassment at my behavior, and am horrified at how gnarled and twisted my mind had become. I knew that I was being a complete bitch, but in my chemically imbalanced mind I felt that my behavior was justified. People who are hurting find release in hurting other people, to be certain.

When I began my journey toward getting help I chose the quickest route possible (apart from being institutionalized), which included an intake therapy appointment at a behavioral health center even though I was already seeing a therapist. I was amazed by the efficiency of that appointment; in under an hour, I was diagnosed with attachment disorder, anxiety disorder, depression (duh), and a myriad of other handy clinical diagnoses; I'm shocked she didn't pull The Book of Crazy from the shelf and start categorically listing all my "isms." From that initial intake appointment, during which I proved to be certifiable enough to move on to the next stage, I was shuffled back to the reception desk to schedule a session with the center's psychiatrist. *Yay, meds!* I felt like a drug addict arriving at a methadone clinic, going through the motions to get my prized prescription for medication that would ease my pain.

Just like my intake therapy experience, the psychiatrist diagnosed me in record time: twenty minutes. In truth, I think I received a speedy diagnosis and prescription because my toddler (who I had to bring to the appointment) and I took turns throwing tearful fits. I left the behavioral health center happily clutching my prescription, which included instructions to consult my OB before I began taking the medication. I didn't like the sound of that; I was still breastfeeding at that time and desperately wanted to get pregnant again, because I wrongly believed getting pregnant would soothe my grief over the miscarriages.

Being the paranoid and inquisitive person that I am, I wanted a second opinion. My distrust of doctors, triggered by mishandling after my first miscarriage, led me to get my second opinion from the ultimate physician: Dr. Internet. I read that the dosage I had been prescribed was likely enough to "tranquilize a bull" and make a vegan eat bacon. Yikes! Ever the armchair doctor and always thinking I knew what was best for me, I foolishly came up with my own dosage plan and began taking my medication every other day. When I finally got in to see the psychiatrist, who coordinated with my therapist, I admitted to self-prescribing my dosage but was flummoxed by the intense headaches and other side effects I was experiencing. Used to seeing nutcases like me on a daily basis, my psychiatrist calmly smiled and began trying to sort out the medication mess I had created. She corrected the dosage for me, insisted that I take it daily and sent me on my way.

Finding my medicinal "sweet spot" was the first hurdle in my journey toward happiness, but mere weeks later I was no longer shouting expletives at drivers who cut me off in traffic, or slowing to five miles under the speed limit when someone chose my bumper to tailgate. Eventually I reached a state of rational calmness that shocked my husband, as episodes that previously would have made me explode no longer fazed me. Dirty laundry dropped next to the hamper no longer infuriated me, and I wasn't reduced to a sobbing mess after a hideous day caring for our toddler.

My husband was so used to walking on eggshells around me that it actually took him a couple months to get used to the new, peaceful me. He approached difficult conversations with his defenses up, often not believing me when I responded in a calm, measured manner.

I know he had to be thinking, *Who is that zen-like woman and what did she do with my wife?!*

These days, I work daily toward achieving a happy, contented state. My mind is no longer at war with itself, and the loop of disparaging messages of self-loathing has finally stopped playing; that's one tape I'm glad got jammed in my personal cassette tape player. Even my psychiatrist has commented on how well I handle my toddler when he gets restless during our bi-monthly check-ins. My response to her is to smile, give an exaggerated wink and say, "Thanks, I'm medicated." My feathers still get ruffled, but it takes much more to knock me off of my happy pedestal.

When the trolls lash out at me online, instead of crying and feeling badly about myself, I vow to mentally throw a parade for all those unhappy people in which I, the Grand Marshal, drive down the street and toss happy pills out to them like candy.

*Lauren B. Stevens is a freelance writer, whose work can also be found on* The Huffington Post, Scary Mommy, *and* Care.com. *When she's not chasing her rambunctious toddler, Lauren can be found blogging about Parenting and Women's Issues on her blog Lo-wren.*

# WHAT BIRTH ANNOUNCEMENTS DON'T SAY

## Noelle Elliott

My friend recently had a baby and bravely shared with me that it wasn't exactly what she had expected—not the birth itself, but the time at home when the visitors taper off, your husband goes back to work and you are alone. In a time when most of my communication with friends happens online, I was a little shocked to receive a phone call. I just listened, because she obviously needed to be heard. I told her I was here for her and hoped that helped. I didn't have time to explain that I knew her pain and isolation.

In 2003, I had my first son. It was great, everybody was happy, but when I got home I had a nagging fear I was going to drop him. Kind of typical really, but my mind didn't just stop there. I would wake up and play the scenario over and over again but in graphic detail. I shared this with a (former) friend who also had a new baby and she told me I was weird. I never mentioned it to my doctor because I figured I was alone and that it was a fleeting thought. It wasn't.

The fear of being labeled insane has kept me from sharing these experiences with many people, but if revealing them helps those like my friend, I will bare my soul. In 2004, my second son was born via a C-section because he was big and breech. I was clueless and ill-prepared for the pain of recovery—until I sneezed.

The six months following his birth were by far the darkest days of my existence. It was a slow, progressive plunge into a place I didn't think my subconscious could take me. I started to have visions of horrific things happening to my baby. For example, I would envision a stranger coming into the house and repeatedly slamming him into the wall, or dropping him on his head. I would think these thoughts in fantastic detail and immediately feel tremendous guilt.

After I decided to take on the job of stay-at-home-mom, I had my hair cut ten inches and dyed it dark brown, trying to look the part. I took pictures, posed with the baby and sent out birth announcements. My husband, Don, knew I wasn't acting like myself, but decided it was due to exhaustion. The combination of having two kids so close together and giving birth in October when sunlight is more limited left me depressed and ragged. He got a glimpse of my true inner turmoil one night when we had an argument. He had gone out with some friends and I thought he would be home sooner. The baby was crying most of the time he was gone and I was slowly losing my mind. By the time he arrived home I was beyond angry and yelled at him. Naturally he was defensive and the verbal sparring began—until I picked up the baby and was poised to throw him up against the wall. I wasn't just threatening, I was about to do it. What happened next will haunt me for ages.

I saw fear in Don's eyes. He slowly approached me and took the baby. I was horrified I had let out what was going on in my head, and that I allowed myself to get so close to the edge. I left. It was eleven at night and I ran. I literally ran, I don't remember how far, but I know it was my sad attempt to run away. I feared going back home. What did he think of me? I begged him to never tell our son what I had said or felt for fear he may feel unwanted.

Don didn't go to work the next day, and whenever he left my mom appeared and vice versa. I started to realize I was never alone with my children, and later I found out it was an arrangement between them. They didn't trust me with myself, or more specifically, with the baby.

I called a doctor and Don went with me to my first appointment. The doctor put me on medication, and reassured my husband I was not going to drown the boys in a bathtub or drive them into a river. He candidly told Don, "Your wife has postpartum anxiety, not postpartum psychosis."

I wasn't convinced.

I was prescribed a heavy antidepressant; I was also instructed to see a therapist every week. The medication stabilized my mind, but I was left with heavy guilt for thinking such horrific thoughts. At the time I failed to realize that hormones are a powerful things and not easily controlled.

In my opinion, the C-section didn't allow my body to recognize that I was having a baby. I never went into labor, and the baby was abruptly removed. It was kind of traumatic for all parties involved, and no one would have known the depth of my illness had Don and I not gotten into that argument. I felt that I had failed, miserably.

I had my third son in 2007. It was in July and to my surprise, even after another C-section, all went well. I could tell my family, however, was leery. My mom would make surprise Starbucks deliveries, or my dad would just happen to be in the neighborhood. There was no need for their concern, though, because this postpartum was medication free.

In 2010 my last son was born. I was doing fine until the actual C-section. I had a panic attack during surgery that lasted into recovery. By the time I could verbalize what was going on, I thought I was going to jump out of my skin. I say panic attack, but it was far worse. I suddenly decided on the operating table to choose flight instead of fight. I wanted to leave and leave now, but when I went to move my legs or arms and I couldn't. I was verbally and physically paralyzed. I could communicate with my eyes and as much as I tried to scream, I couldn't. The surgery went on. I tried to sing in my head to muffle the doctor's voices. The following night my mind gave me a glimpse of what I had feared, the depression coming again. I didn't want to admit it; I had done so well last time. I didn't tell Don, but I didn't want to be alone.

Despite me asking, pleading with him to stay, he left at 11:00 p.m. and said he would be back at 7:00 a.m. with a latte and a bagel (our post-birth tradition).

Around the time Don left, they brought the baby in so I could feed him. When I was finished I called the nurse and asked her to come take him back the nursery. I was scared, and didn't want to let my mind go to that place, but it did. I panicked. I called Don, told him I couldn't do this, and hung up. I looked at the baby in the little, clear bassinet and horrific thoughts came rushing to my head. Where was the nurse? I tried to call again. What was taking so long? I locked myself in the bathroom until I heard them come in.

Tears were running down my face, and I explained I needed to see a doctor. The nurse asked if I was in pain. I told her I was, but not physically. They told me the soonest a doctor could see me would be in the morning. I paced back and forth. She took the baby to the nursery as Don was walking in.

I asked him to never ask me what was going on in my head, but to forgive me. I also thanked him for being there. That night was a long one. In the morning a doctor arrived. Don was in the room when he asked me to tell him what thoughts I was having. I figured if he had been with me despite my flawed maternal issues, he wasn't going to leave now, so I spoke plainly and calmly about how I wanted to hurt our baby. I felt exposed. *Not again*, I thought. After a long pause the doctor spoke without alarm in his voice. He looked me in the eyes and said something that got me through the next six months. He said, "Allow those thoughts to come into your mind, acknowledge them, and dismiss them. Find comfort in knowing that you have a pure conscience and you would never harm your baby."

Perhaps it was the combination of the drugs and the fact my doctor didn't look at me like I was crazy, but I can confidently say I came out ahead. I found immense comfort in neighbors, family and friends bringing dinner over, and socializing, even if it was brief and they didn't have a clue what I was going through.

To my friend and any mother experiencing this same trauma, I'll tell you this: Although you may be feeling overwhelmed, scared, disappointed, guilty, know that you are a good mom. You will overcome this and I have confidence in your pure conscience that you will climb out of this dark place. Don't define yourself by a stereotypical mom that only exists on a feel-good sitcom, or assume other moms have it all together. Up until now, you thought I did.

*Noelle lives in the Midwest where she works in publicity at a university. She is a contributing writer for* Family and Sassy *magazines and has been featured on several websites including* Elephant Journal, Yahoo, Erma Bombeck *and* Tabata Times. *She is a contributing writer at* In The Powder Room. *She is the creator of the acclaimed staged production* The Mamalogues, Dramas from Real Mamas. *Noelle is the force behind the blog* Bow Chica Bow Mom, *where she writes about her lofty mission to raise the next generation of gentleman.*

# THE WAVES OF MY LIFE

## Lance Burson

The first time someone called me crazy, I was twelve years old.
I'm a classic overachiever who started young. I spent the early part of the 1980s as the smallest and youngest boy in my class. The only ways I knew to deal with bullying were sharp wit and the occasional freak out. But as any comedian will tell you, the funny isn't something you can just pull out of your backpack between science and math class to fend off someone six inches taller who wants to take out the anguish of their parents' divorce on your scrawny butt.

Four years later, at age sixteen, I was diagnosed with anxiety and depression. I was smart but my grades were suffering and I'd started drinking to placate the internal demons that continually strangled me. I became a regular on the high school party scene, lied to my parents about where I was in order to get access to alcohol, and kept bottles hidden in my room or near the creek behind my family's house.

Only the crazy people in suburban Atlanta in 1986 saw a shrink—not a teenage kid with some issues. I was unprepared to take on the stigma of being medicated so instead I drank, and did the best I could over the next two decades. I struck up a long-term love affair with alcohol. It has played as much a part in my life as my relationships have, sometimes even more. Alcohol medicated my mental illness for over twenty years.

I had finally had enough when I was thirty-six years old. It was Thanksgiving, and I wasn't thankful. Instead I was lost, resigned, and alone. I packed two bags and wrote a goodbye letter, which I left on the kitchen counter of the house I was renting from my family. I hoped they would come by unexpectedly, without calling, and find the note. It was my insurance policy, of sorts, pushing me over the edge of the cliff I was hanging from. I didn't think they'd even try to find me but if so, I'd be gone, very gone, by then.

Two months earlier I'd sat in divorce court and watched whom I was die. When the judge rendered her decision, I left that person behind and wandered aimlessly, disconnected, for weeks. I was now divorced and reduced to seeing my daughter less than half the time. I was again the black sheep of my family, a sad, thirty-six-year-old man in the grip of a midlife crisis and in debt. In an effort to escape my world I accepted an offer from a longtime friend to spend the Thanksgiving holiday in Key West and do as Ernest Hemingway did when he resided there: drink.

The day I left for the Keys, my friend called and said he couldn't make the trip. The person I left in the courtroom months earlier would have unpacked his bags, felt sorry for his loneliness, and sulked until something ridiculous came along to distract him. The purgatory me got in my car, and drove thirteen hours.

I stopped at a gas station near the beach in Miami. While the car was filling up, I walked a hundred yards and stood in the middle of the shore and contemplated staying there or going back home. Then I made a new plan, one that almost ended me. I kept going.

When I made it to the Keys, the motel shanty I chose for its low price was pathetic looking. It was dingy and unkempt. The screen door was broken. Outside, on the tiniest patio you could imagine, sat a grill that had seen better days. The entire place was a parallel to my life. But the beach was only thirty feet away. It was a postcard for a last stand.

Two days later, Thanksgiving came. My feast was one grilled, medium rare steak. Apropos of my zombie state. I ate and watched the waves roll in, the sound calming my anxiousness. By my third beer, I decided to walk the thirty feet and try the cold ocean water despite the 55-degree temperature. Before I reached the tide line, I noticed how warm the sand was, so I removed my shoes and socks. I sat down on the berm, reached my hand out and felt the texture of the tan grains. I had a beer in my left hand and poured a tiny amount into the sand. I ran the grains of sand over the wet spot. The symbolism made me smile for the first time in two months. I let go.

The twenty years of drinking and abuse of my body and mind had left me at a point where I wanted to stop. What stop meant was open to interpretation, even to myself. I thought about all the friends, girlfriends, and now a wife that had come and gone. **I was good at getting** them but bad at keeping them. I'd even managed to marry someone with the same issues I had. Along the path, we squeezed the birth of my daughter into the chaos. The divorce that followed, and sent me to my moment on the beach, was the lowest point of my life.

I sat on the Key West beach, watching the water run over the sand as my mental state unraveled. I thought about one of the most profound moments of my life. It was just a few months earlier, in February 2006. I was thirty-five years old, in a therapist's office for the first time. It was forty-eight steps from my car to the door of the office. I counted them each of the four times I made the walk before going inside. No one I knew went to a professional, yet there I was, doing so, without encouragement or support. Thinking of my therapist, of those forty-eight steps, must have helped me that day because I made it off the beach when the possibility of not making it was very real.

I tried to end my life but I didn't. I lowered my body into the water. It rose above my head and I took water into my lungs. Something happened, I can't explain, but what I wanted to happen did not and suddenly I felt myself above the surface gasping for air. I walked out of the water and sat on the beach, ashamed of myself. The sense of failure was overwhelming but I focused on my three year old daughter and drank in the margins of time when we weren't together. I would go through the motions, do the things on the surface that seemed like things a good parent would do, but I was too far down, and had so much work to do.

Over the next several days, weeks and months, I changed my life into something I could live with, something better. I started working on myself. I listened to my therapist, I read books, I found support online and off. The right diagnosis and medication followed. Then I got a second chance at everything. Through the help of the woman I married two years later in 2008, along with two new daughters, I blended my family into five. I got better, and I stopped drinking. Being the father to three girls and a husband to someone who actually loved me and encouraged me to work on myself held me to a higher standard. Each day is a struggle but instead of booze to get me through, I have them, and a greater purpose.

Writing has meant as much to me as pills or therapy. The four women I live with have cheered me on to realize my dream of being a published writer.

It's been eight years since I lost hope. I've rediscovered it through the people around me. At forty-four years old I feel like a teenager again, mentally. But, tomorrow could be different. I need to be ready.

Bipolar disorder isn't a death sentence, but it is a life sentence. How I do the time has changed. I have evolved thanks to the right diagnosis, medication, and support. Now it's possible to go to the beach and just have fun.

*Lance Burson is a writer living in Atlanta, Georgia with his wife and three daughters and not taking about Fight C..... He's the published author of 2 books,* The Ballad Of Helene Troy *and* Soul To Body, *available on Amazon and in paperback through Lulu.com. You can follow Lance and all his wit on his blog, Lance My Blog Can Beat Up Your Blog.*

# EVERYBODY POOPS—
# INCLUDING THE NEIGHBORS

## Kathryn Leehane

*Author's Note: Sometimes talking about mental illness is like sharing a private moment. It can be awkward, uncomfortable, and just plain shitty. I really wish it wasn't, and much like poop, I'll talk about mental illness until it becomes a norm.*

I often hear my fellow moms say they want to go to the bathroom alone, that they want some privacy when nature calls. Honestly, I can't really relate to this at all. I've never had that wish.

Because I've never gone to the bathroom alone. Not in my entire life.

Growing up in a large family, I shared a bathroom with my six siblings. To speed up throughput, my mom installed saloon-style doors to separate the toilet and shower area from the sink and mirror area. (Genius move, if you ask me.) Still, while the doors may have created some visual privacy, they did nothing to dampen the, erm, sounds from the toilet. What I'm saying is that we heard everything going on with everybody. Everything.

It didn't take long for me to realize that if I wanted any time in the bathroom truly to myself, I either had to get up really early or stay up really late. I've always prized sleep, so neither one of those alternatives worked for me. Instead, I quickly learned to just let it go no matter who was nearby. Otherwise, I would have suffered many an accident on the floor. Or my bladder would have exploded.

My sister and I even had an agreement that one of us could use the toilet if the other one was in the shower—modesty be damned. Let's face it, at that point there was no line I wouldn't cross in order to use the piss pot. (Although we did try to avoid number two. Even the best smelling soaps can't cover up a post-bean-burrito dump.)

Long story short, the concept of bathroom privacy has never existed for me.

In high school I spent the summers living and working at a campground outside of Yosemite that had dormitory-style bathrooms. We were a little wilder and a little more free there, so no one really cared that much. One of my best friends and I even made up a bathroom song (based on a church song, naturally) for when we were sitting next to each other in the stalls:

*My pee is flowing like a river*
*Flowing out of you and me*
*Flowing out into the sewer*
*Setting all the bladders free.*

I'll spare you the verse for poop. You're welcome.

When I got to college, we had co-ed dormitories. Which also meant we had co-ed bathrooms, and a co-ed audience to any and all evacuations. There was literally no alternative to pooping within earshot of said co-ed audience, but unlike some people, I really wasn't all that bothered by it. Honestly, it wasn't much different than my house growing up. And I wasn't about to miss my window of opportunity by holding it in.

This philosophy carried me into my adult years. When my husband and I were still dating, we took a trip to Lake Tahoe with some friends. After indulging in too many bacon-wrapped filet mignons at the casino buffet, I excused myself to use the toilet. As the liquid horror poured from my ass, and as a sound like someone angrily kick-starting a Harley Davidson echoed throughout the bathroom, the other women in the vicinity were effectively silenced. I didn't really care, but clearly I was making them uncomfortable.

Outside of the facilities, my husband and his friend waited for me as a line of appalled women walked out of the bathroom.

Horrified women streamed past, simultaneously exclaiming, "Oh. My. Gawd!"

My husband and friend both knew, "That must be Kate."

These are things I'm used to. However, my poor husband was not.

When we got married, there wasn't any privacy in our one-bathroom apartment. This didn't faze me, but my husband had some trouble adjusting.

Me (through the bathroom door): "Hey, what do you want for dinner?"

Husband (from the porcelain throne): "Uhhhh, could we talk about this later?"

Me: "Why? You're free right now."

Husband: —

Me: "Okay, fine. We'll talk when you're done pooping."

Husband: "Thank you. 'Cuz, really?"

Me: "Everybody poops, Tim."

Our cats learned quickly that someone in the bathroom was stationary and available for head scratches. They would come in to get their fill. They had no pride. They didn't care if I was shit-petting them.

And once we got dogs, there was a whole new level of interaction in the bathroom. Dogs are like, "Oh, hey! What you doing?" "Oh, hey! What's that smell?" "Oh, hey! Did you step on a frog?" They even learned to bring me the ball so we could play fetch from the toilet.

Multitasking, people.

So when I had kids, it was no big deal to take them with me into the bathroom. Or to have them come in because they wanted to hang out. I've signed report cards on the toilet. I've put on my son's neck gear. (Don't worry—this was pre-wiping, folks. I'm not unsanitary.) I've had deep discussions about which boys at school are cute, and I've helped my daughter pick out which shoes go best with her outfit. I'm not saying that I love doing this with my kids around. But I'm used to it. When you gotta go, you gotta go. It's just life.

Because I've gotten so used to animals and kids being with me in the bathroom, I just leave the bathroom door open all of the time. (Energy conservation. Seriously.) So this happens a lot:

Husband (walking into the bedroom): "Where's the [insert any easily located item from my house]? Oh, sorry. You're on the toilet."

Me: "No problem. It's in the—"

Husband: "I'll ask later. Close the door."

Me: "What?! I'm only pooping."

Husband: "Where's the line, Kate? Close the door!"

Me: "Everybody poops, Tim."

Husband: —

I wish R.E.M. sang about that instead.

I was recently at a conference where all attendees were staying in a college dorm, with dormitory bathrooms. Of course, I didn't even think twice about it. When some of the women expressed their fear of public pooping, I promised to do my loudest impression of Ethel Merman singing "Welcome to the Jungle" to drown out any noises. I don't understand why no one took me up on the offer.

So we've established I'm pretty lackadaisical when it comes to pooping in front of other people. I even have an unofficial Poop Club with two of my friends in which we text each other after we've pooped. (I think I just broke the first rule of Poop Club.) We congratulate each other much like you might congratulate a child in the midst of potty-training. Sometimes we even send each other selfies while on the toilet. Yeah. I know. Not everyone gets it. My husband being one of them. He remains horrified by all discussions of pooping.

Don't worry. I remember to close the bathroom door when company comes over. Most of the time. I do know where the line is.

At least I thought I did.

Last summer, our street was having a block party. It was later in the evening, and I really had to pee. Since our house is way down on the corner (and I'm super lazy), I asked my neighbor if I could use her bathroom. Naturally she said yes.

I went inside their house and over to the bathroom. I knocked softly on the door. Nothing. I tried the handle. Unlocked. So I opened the door only to walk in on my neighbor's husband.

Pants down.

Taking a shit. (While reading *Popular Mechanics*.)

That article must have been very engrossing, because I guess he didn't hear me knock. But he sure heard the door open.

"Uh, this is occupied!" he stammered as I walked in the room.

My jaw dropped, and I froze. "Oh, fuck. I'm sorry."

I turned around and left the bathroom faster than, well, as fast as someone who just walked in on her neighbor's husband taking a shit. I haven't spoken to him since. Or looked him in the eye. Or read *Popular Mechanics*. (Not that I have ever read it in the first place.)

I guess we found our definitive line that day. But you know what? I can't help but wonder if we could have avoided the whole mess had he kept the door open.

*Kathryn Leehane is a writer and humorist living in the San Francisco Bay Area with her husband and two children. Along with inhaling books, bacon and Pinot Noir, she writes the humor blog,* Foxy Wine Pocket, *where she shares twisted (and only sometimes exaggerated and inappropriate) stories about her life as a mother, wife, friend and wine-drinker in suburbia. She is a contributing author to several anthologies and is at work on her first book--a memoir about loss and survival. Her essays have also been featured on* BLUNTmoms, The Huffington Post, Mamapedia, Megsanity, Scary Mommy, *and more.*

# ALONE ON AN ISLAND OF MISFIT TOYS

## Audrey Hayworth

I've had issues all my life, as far back as I can remember. It started with chronic sexual abuse by a male relative and a sexual assault, which marred my life in a way that could make the hardest heart ache for my story. These moments, however, also triggered the beginning of a thirty-year struggle within my own mind.

The sexual abuse started when I was a young child; by the age of seven I hated my changing body. Academic journals will tell you this is textbook behavior for a female who has been abused. Before puberty, I took comfort in the fact that I could feel my bones and obsessively counted the number of ribs on my ribcage.

So, unbeknownst to my parents, around the age of seven I began to cut snacks out of my diet. I recorded this day in my diary, declaring I no longer wanted to be fat. I meticulously watched what I ate, and every night when I would lie in bed, I made sure I could still feel my hipbones sticking out.

This behavior went on for years, and I showed the classic signs of depression: school suffered, I was moody, and I slept for many hours at a time. When I was fourteen, my parents found out what was really going on with me—I was being sexually abused and as a result I had developed anorexia nervosa.

The floor below me seemed to crumble under the weight of this revelation and my only source of control, food, was suddenly on everyone's radar. Weigh-ins, doctors' visits, psychiatry and therapy visits became a daily routine for two years.

The eating disorder got worse, it seemed, instead of better, once the food came under their control and not my own. My hair started to fall out, and I developed a very fine hair on my body called lanugo. Once the doctors finally found a medication that helped subside the obsessive thoughts I had about gaining weight and dull the depressive thoughts I was able to gain weight and come to a healthy BMI. I was finally stable.

That is, until my seventeenth birthday, when I was raped. The stability that I knew only fleetingly was gone, and nothing, absolutely nothing mattered to me for a long time. My weight plummeted; at my lowest I weighed seventy-two pounds that year.

⇒⁺ ⁺⇐

Looking back, it is hard to believe such short snippets of time have dictated my emotional state for the last twenty years. But it is our collective experience that shapes us and our brains, and for better or for worse, they are our own stories.

Years of therapy passed, and I slowly began to understand there are good people in this world, not just evil. And yet, this dark cloud hung over me at all times. I still obsessed about my weight.

Depression is the shadow of an eating disorder. For the longest time, I was told the depression was "situational," a direct product of anorexia. But what happens when the "situational depression" becomes the actual situation? I've learned there is an ebb and flow to all things related to my darker moods. Seasons, weather, children, jobs, health—they all play into the episodes of depression.

When I was younger, I felt so different and alone in this cycle of self-hatred and loathing. It felt, and still does to an extent, as if I am watching the world with my nose pressed to the window pane of life, the happy people basking in the light on the inside, and me alone on the island of misfit toys, outside in the dark.

That's the thing about depression—it taints everything I do. It aches and perceives truths in ways I know not to be true, leaving me unable to trust my own mind. I survive in the shadows, through tinted lenses of life. It sucks me into its vacuumed vortex, and only by clawing my way out of its tunnel does it seem I can survive. I am left feeling different, bruised and damaged. The truth is, I am different, but by no means am I alone.

Therapy and medicine have gotten me to the point where I see my depression and anorexia for what they are: mental disorders that are a part of my story. Because no matter how many years pass, food and the number on the scale are still the first things that come to my mind the moment I wake up. I can never say I am cured, because I will be in recovery my whole life. The more my life is out of control, the more I will strive to control the scale. This is my truth. The ugly, miserable truth in a dark recessed part of my mind.

This truth also includes the fact that depression will most likely never leave me. That no matter how much I talk about what happened to me, how many hours I talk to therapists, how many magic pills I try, nothing will fix that part of my brain. The trauma of my life is there, playing like a broken record on repeat in the back of my mind, haunting my days and encroaching into my nightmares. My heart is heavy, and yet, at the same time hopeful that one day the broken record will play a little less, and the number on the scale will be enough to satisfy me. Because really, sometimes hope is all I have at the end of the day—and hope is enough for me to want to see another day.

*Audrey Hayworth is a redheaded, mother of two boys and a Southern transplant. She lives in Baton Rouge, Louisiana where the best things in life can be found: family, friends, food, and an international airport within 30 minutes. While most days she considers it a success to shower and not let the kids burn the house down she also finds time to blog on her site* Sass Mouth *where she waxes and wanes about the challenging, embarrassing, and magical life of raising two autistic boys (one serious, one a dimpled lunatic), throwing parties, attempting to do all things that a 'good' Southern lady would do, all while trying to make the world a better place.*

# I WANT TO SCREAM

## Zoe Lewis

I want to scream so loud and hard that my voice box explodes and my eyes pop out. I want to scream in such a way that the vibrations would cause tectonic plates to shift, enormous undulating screams that would reverberate through the universe and shift the pattern of space and time. God damn it! I want to scream.

I know I'm not alone in this. For instance, at this very moment my freshly minted two-year-old daughter is doing a truly magnificent job of screaming. She's howling at me with such rage and ever-increasing pitch, that surely she is communicating with another species. I fear a pod of dolphins has started to amass off the coastline and is planning a coup. The injustices of life, kid—they're a bitter pill to swallow. It's all about perspective.

Perspective is an odd thing. Take away all the material bullshit of life and what are you left with? The one thing you can control is your-self, isn't it? What happens when that control gets taken away? We can whine that we don't have this gadget or those toys, that vacation or live in this neighborhood, but all of it gets put into stark perspective when you can't control your own body or mind.

It started off so imperceptibly that I barely noticed it. There were frequent headaches (who doesn't get those?), random aches and pains in various parts of my body. I rationalized it was my ripe old age of thirty; we're all getting older, nothing to worry about.

But then I lost time. Ever done that? I'd take a moment, blink, and an hour had passed, an hour for which I had no memory. Entire conversations vanished from my recollection. Surely, it happens to us all, doesn't it?

Then there was the insomnia. Insomnia? God, we've all had that.

I had so many minor problems that I felt foolish bringing them up. Individually they could be dismissed. I placated my apprehension, convinced myself that all people experience these things.

But slowly the issues started getting out control. I wouldn't sleep for days on end, existing on a series of naps. My mind would torture me by night with endless to do, have I done, or should I do lists. Whichever current annoying song was played constantly on the radio would get stuck in my head on a loop. Over and over it would play, and not even the whole damn song. Just part of it. I wanted to drive a fork into my brain for some peace. I was becoming more than slightly irrational. I was hypersensitive and panicky. Simple decisions and actions became impossible. *It must be hormones,* I thought.

Except my body hurt so much that I would shuffle out of bed in the morning like an octogenarian. The slightest poke felt like someone had just punched me, but I felt like a hypochondriac for even mentioning it. So many random, seemingly unrelated annoyances had silently taken over my life. *Suck it up missy, nobody cares.* There was nothing visibly wrong with me, so I must have been an attention seeker.

The first diagnosis came in my early thirties. Depressed—Christ, who isn't? Next up, borderline personality disorder with avoidant tendencies. Huh, well there you go. Sounded like I was going to go all Britney Spears and shave my head and shit. Then came ADD. This was not a shocker, and somewhat of a relief. The thing was, the diagnoses didn't stop there.

Along with the crazy-town side, there were a multitude of physiological problems. A litany of specialists and quacks from every specialty had an opinion. I was poked, prodded tested and violated in every conceivable way. The results were: fibromyalgia, hypermobility, chronic pain syndrome, restless leg syndrome, and so very much more. There were syndromes and disorders up and out the yin-yang. My life was summed up in a veritable laundry list of illnesses, syndromes, disorders and diseases. Each had its turn as the diagnosis de jour.

I was overwhelmed. I was drowning in a pit of my own misery and pain. It all seemed enormous and uncontrollable. How in the hell could I find my way out from all of it?

The one thing I was never diagnosed with was being a stubborn bitch, but if restless leg syndrome is a thing then so is stubborn bitch syndrome. I am the most pig-headed person in the world, and that's a good thing. I wallowed for a while, comfortable in the knowledge that I had a medical reason for malingering. A medical *condition,* no less. I was told to "give myself a break" or "allow myself to feel." *Fuck off!* My pity party didn't last long.

I fought off despair when I stopped seeing the whole and started seeing pieces. What could I manage today? Instead of treating an entire disorder or syndrome as a whole, why not just deal with what is happening right now? Later is later. Every small step was a win. Get up in the morning? It's a win. Make the bed? Another win. My days became a series of small battles, fought but not always won.

I hold myself to ridiculously high standards and I know it. But if you have the energy to complain, then you have the energy to start helping yourself. I had no idea how to do that though, so I had to swallow my pride and ego and get professional help. I had to inform those closest to me of my problem. Some didn't get it. Some still don't. Those who did, like my husband, have been my rock. On my crazy days, when I can't think straight or when I can barely walk, he is there. I truly expected him to turn around and run for the hills, as I am sure as shit not low maintenance, but he didn't.

Friends help, too. They get it when I don't make it to functions or a night out. These are friends who also call me on my bullshit when I am being a stubborn asshole. I had to ask for allowances and it killed me, but in doing so I also discovered I wasn't alone. There are lots of us out there in crazy town, struggling through life one symptom or syndrome at a time.

My life is smaller now. It took me a long time to be happy with that, to learn that smaller is not less than, it's just smaller and more manageable. I get it wrong as often as I get it right. There are days when I feel like Wonder Woman, complete with gold tiara, bustier, and star spangled knickers (I actually have those), and I do too much only to have my ass kicked later by my resentful body. There are days when I struggle to get out bed and put one foot in front of the other. I take each day with each battle as they come. You win some and you lose some, but if I can make it to the end of the day without sucking down a shit load of pain killers then it's a win. If my kid is fed, clean(ish), and I didn't punch an annoying person in the face, it's a win.

We all have days when we want to scream at the kids for being the destructive little shits that they are, and I am no exception. We all have days when we pray for sweet release from the endless headache-inducing tirade of bullshit, bodily fluids, bills, and minutiae that make us crazy.

I am not alone and this gives me comfort. I may not scream out loud, as this invariably gives me a headache and is somewhat counterproductive, but I am allowed to scream. We all have problems and perspective is not always an attractive truth (especially when provided by someone else); but as I listen now to the silence, I know the small ball of raging snot screaming at me from her prison (bed) has finally fallen asleep. I have had my hour to write this and breathe.

It's a lot more than some people get. The urge to scream has left me. Perspective is an amazing thing isn't it?

*Zoë is an English woman living in the Netherlands with her Dutch husband, a lethargic Spanish greyhound and a Machiavellian toddler. Lewis is out to prove that the mums that create Pinterest worthy bento lunchboxes or adorable hand-sewn toddler outfits in the space of a 40-minute nap are dirty liars. Come on over to her blog George with Ears for the eye rolling grammatical fails and stay for the crappy Instagram photography, and her latest illustrations.*

# CLASS DISMISSED
## Tammy Rutledge

I was going through a bitter divorce when I first started learning to drive a school bus. The career kind of chose me, as I was suddenly without daycare and needed a kid-friendly source of income. Plus, I loved to drive and relished the challenge of driving a huge vehicle. At least, I relished the challenge until the first time I drove a huge vehicle. Then I was terrified, but committed to giving it my best shot for my son's sake, and because I felt I had something to prove as a woman behind the wheel.

It was my first day driving, and training consisted of a few of us going out in a bus with the trainer and taking turns driving in traffic to demonstrate what we were capable of. I couldn't do much other than drive straight, and the look on the trainer's face as he whipped his head around and over his shoulder to see if I was going to take the pole down as I skirted around the corner, oblivious to the mechanics of bus driving, was unforgettable. I missed the light pole, but barely. He removed me from the driver's seat and provided lessons in a parking lot after that.

Somehow, after a gazillion hours of practical training, countless written tests, and an excruciating road test, I got my license to drive a bus one sunny, crisp September morning. That same afternoon I was sent on my first bus run all by myself. It was a special route, reserved for drivers that had just passed their road test. It was through a newly developed (and in some areas still being built) neighborhood. As if I wasn't nervous enough, my route sheet had roads on it that didn't even exist! It was the last informal test and fortunately the kids were accustomed to the route and the routine of a new driver. They were kind enough to give accurate directions when the sheet failed me.

At the prompting of my passengers, I headed down a street that was divided with pylons in the middle; my side of the road was new pavement while the other side was freshly ripped up into grooves. I probably went two or three kilometers before I came to a group of construction workers. As I approached in my bus, I saw their faces drop and then turn to shock. They started waving frantically at me to get off my side of the road. This is when it occurred to me that I should check my rear-view. I was stunned to see I was driving my bus down freshly laid pavement! Even though the construction crew should have had that side of the road closed off with a barricade, I was certain I was to blame and was going to be fired on my first official day. I went home and tried not to panic or burst into flames from the embarrassment. The bus gods must have been smiling on me that day, because I never heard so much as a whisper about my sticky situation.

The next day, my second official day driving a school bus, I started the run I would drive for the next four years. I was assigned to transport seventh- and eighth-grade students exclusively. I was driving in an old residential neighborhood with very narrow roads. I hugged the curb too tightly as I headed downhill and around a curve to the right, and that damn tail swing caught the curb ever so slightly. The right hand side of the bus jumped unexpectedly as if I had hit a speed bump, triggering one of the students to swear at me, ask me who taught me to drive, and then start to proclaim she wanted her old bus driver back. The bus gods intervened again, because before she could even finish her sentence she was smacked right in the face by a run-away rogue tree branch. I was still too close to the curb, and the ancient overgrown trees were reaching into the open windows. After it smacked her in the face and effectively silenced her mid-sentence, it proceeded to smack the kids in the two seats behind her for good measure. I pulled a little further from the curb, and delivered incredibly quiet students to school that morning without further comments or incidents. Again, I was terrified I was going to lose my job, but it turns out that grade seven and eight students don't tell their parents a whole lot about their day.

After those two incidents I drove without anything out of the ordinary occurring for years and years, other than being t-boned by a dude trying to cut across four lanes to make a left hand turn. He said he didn't see me and tried to convince the officer that I snuck up on him while traveling at 40 kilometers an hour down a straight, unoccupied road in a bright yellow, 70-passenger school bus. I'm pretty sure he got charged. I've always wondered what his wife had to say when he tried to convince her that he encountered a very sneaky school bus and totaled his rather new looking minivan.

The only thing I didn't really like about driving the bus was fueling it up. I felt a great deal of anxiety maneuvering such a large vehicle around gas pumps, and I hated how long it took to fill up in bad weather. One particular day I was in a hurry because I had class at the local university that evening, so I set the pump to automatically fill the tank while I went about cleaning all the windows. I had just started school so I was wearing my best jeans and one of my nicest tops, hoping not to feel too out of place among students who were half-dozen years younger than I was. As I circled the bus to clean the windows, I tried to step over the gas hose but the tip of my boot caught it and yanked the nozzle out of the bus while it was still set to auto-fill. Now, industrial gas pumps pump gas a whole lot faster than your local gas station. I instantly found myself being showered with diesel as the hose supported itself and danced around on the ground, shooting fuel straight up over my head. Everybody laughed at me. I couldn't help but laugh, too. Bonus: after my gasoline shower, the station removed the auto-fill feature. I guess the bus gods did have to get me back after all; that's okay, I'll take a gasoline shower over unemployment any day.

While none of my newbie incidents seemed funny at the time, I've found myself looking back and laughing at them. I remind myself that winners never quit and quitters never win. We are all new to something at some point and someone somewhere is trying to achieve something for the very first time. I try to give myself a bit of grace in those moments. And if I ever see someone covered in diesel, I don't laugh too loud. I do try to always carry a clean set of clothes, though, because you just never know when you will need it.

*Tammy Rutledge is a Mother to 3 boys and a boat load of dogs. She earned a degree in Psychology with a minor in Sociology after starting her beautiful family. In her rare spare moments she's finding her voice on her blog,* Daze by Crazy, *and is happily exploring the blogosphere and all the wonderful things it has to offer.*

# FINDING RELIEF
# IN DIAGNOSIS
## Barbara Trainin Blank

When someone like Robin Williams dies by his own hand, or Philip Seymour Hoffman from an apparent drug overdose, people speak about the waste of it all. They wring their hands and pay temporary attention to depression, bipolar illness, and to the substance abuse that sometimes accompanies them in the mentally ill person's attempt to self-medicate. Then the interest passes, along with the intensity of the mourning. Until the next celebrity.

Mood disorders and sometimes self-destructive behavior of famous creative people hit me a little harder and longer than they probably do most people. I've been aware of the torment of mental illness (and especially of mood disorders, such as depression and manic depression, the older term for bipolar illness) since childhood, though I couldn't always put a word or diagnosis to it. I went through many moments of oversensitivity in response to perceived rejection, and many down moods as a kid.

I made a pseudo-suicide attempt (jumping off a balcony not high enough to do anything more than break bones and ruin part of my college career) at age twenty. At about twenty-three, I made a real attempt—pills, from which I miraculously awakened after a few days. Whenever a passing, fleeting thought of suicide takes hold of me, I remind myself that I have been there, done that, and not successfully. So I'd best take another course.

But no one had ever placed a label of mental illness or mood disorder on me. Not until 1980—some eleven years after my jump. That kind of surprised me, considering that my maternal grandfather had been hospitalized for depression shortly before his death. In fact, it masked the cancer that killed him. Back in those days, the 1950s, there were no antidepressants, and virtually no drug therapy except for anxiety. He underwent the old-school type of electroconvulsive shock, which had a positive effect controlling his depression, despite sounding like torture.

Looking back I'm convinced he was bipolar rather than a unipolar depressive. Maybe it was just suggestive: he was creative, an artist who also played musical instruments and could be, my mother said, "the life of the party."

I think, also in retrospect, that my father was cyclothymic, a milder version of bipolar. And it certainly sounds as if his father was given to moods and fits of temper. Yet my father had tremendous energy and talent. It's all in the family, for me.

When I was growing up, therapists and everyone else knew I was given to bad moods, which weren't even called depression, necessarily. They also knew what the precipitating cause was (other than from chemistry and genetics, which people were less likely to speak of then). It was a feeling of rejection, most specifically by men. The men I mourned had some feelings for me, but not to the extent that I had for them, which was more frustrating and painful than if they had none at all. The sense of rejection, combined with my low self-esteem (sometimes alternating with a high opinion of myself) conspired to create an intractable depression.

There were other times when I was up, motivated by creativity or by love or infatuation. When I was a young adult, no one spoke to me about manic depression, something I first learned of in college psychology courses. But a close friend of a guy I was dating in the 1970s commented that I reminded him of a peacock. He accused me of doing everything in an exaggerated fashion, whether it was highs or lows. Much as I disliked the guy, his remark became useful when I considered the bipolar diagnosis pinned on me with assurance about fifteen years later.

One instance of infatuation gone wrong was in 1980. I had been hit by not one, or two, but three romantic disappointments in the two previous years. One was the rejection by a man I had loved as a teenager who came back to me through twisted circumstances. He was really the first person I was in love with, and his disappearance a second time crushed me. I became depressed and obsessive for months, driving my friends crazy as I talked about him over and over. A few months later, though, I met someone else, with whom I was happy and felt optimistic. When he too left my life, I became depressed for a while, but then it lifted. That seemed like real emotional progress. Wrong! The reason the depression was lifting was that, for the first time ever, I was morphing into psychotic mania.

Unfortunately, nobody caught it. At least not until the very end, when some people I spent time with, not even close friends, noticed my tell-tale sign of "pressured speech" where I jumped from one topic to another, cutting everyone else off.

The psychiatrist I was seeing didn't notice it either. He was giving me antidepressants, and one in particular had a tendency to make me feel high. Of course, he didn't know I was bipolar at the time, but my mother still wanted to sue him. The real beef I had against him was that the day I showed up for my appointment and told him I "didn't need therapy anymore," he just shrugged and accepted it. Didn't question it. Didn't call anyone in the family. It was just such an uncharacteristic thing for me to say, and he should have done something. It's hard going for help when your therapist isn't giving you what you need.

It was also in 1980 that I had recently moved to Queens (my parents were in Manhattan at the time), which didn't help matters any. I didn't know anyone there. I was out of work, doing meager amounts of freelance to scrape by. Soon I wasn't sleeping and hardly eating, though I was neither tired nor hungry. I began to hear voices. They didn't tell me to do anything harmful—not to anyone else. The voices were only bizarre and destructive for me. One cold, windy day in December, I went out by myself wearing only a thin raincoat on top of a slip. A dangerous gamble because I was new to the neighborhood and it was nighttime, I'm not sure how I found my way back but I assume the voices led me. I remain amazed I didn't contract pneumonia, or worse, along with mania.

These same voices told me to walk down a particular street in a rather insistent way and to run all around the city between appointments. I was already twenty pounds thinner as a result of my mental illness, and I didn't need to expend extra calories on a manic marathon.

The voices urged me to write a novel, in three languages, all in a week—after the mania had evaporated, I threw it away in my parents' compactor, dismissing it as "crazy."

The voices exhorted me to give away nearly all my money to beggars or others who looked needy on the street. I subsisted on one tuna can divided into three parts for meals because I had virtually nothing to live on.

These same voices told me later to shed all my clothing and lie in my parents' basement, in the laundry room, waiting for my "groom." I didn't have a boyfriend at the time, though I did have a fantasy that the last guy who had broken up with me was coming back. It is of no surprise that I ended up in the psychiatric ward of a hospital.

The undressing was all part of the hypersexuality that sometimes accompanies mania, though there was probably more to it than that. Normally modest, even when undressing in camp or the school locker room in front of other girls, and averse to bad language, I found myself undressing again in the hospital in front of staff and cursing out my completely baffled mother. I had never said a mean, vulgar thing to her before, and haven't since.

The in-house psychiatric staff wasn't sure what to make of what I was going through. They guessed at "reactive psychosis" (a burst of psychotic behavior that occurs when stressed). I later found out that many bipolar patients are originally diagnosed with something else, often schizophrenia. But, *just in case,* they gave me lithium, which helped.

After a period of some noncompliance and another major romantic breakup, I became quite manic, even more than the first time, and ended up in the hospital again five years later.

This time, they were sure.

I remember my father being very troubled by the bipolar label, as if the label were more disturbing than the disease. I, however, was thrilled. It explained many things—the moods, the suicide attempts, the heightened romantic and sexual feelings, even my predilection for buying in thrift shops. Once there was a diagnosis there could be, if not a cure, then a treatment plan. I've been on medication ever since. Life is not perfect, and neither is the control over my moods. But I feel like a person closer to normal than ever before. Someone who is able to love and work, to use Freud's paradigm, however imperfectly. And that is worth quite a lot.

*Barbara Trainin Blank is an award-winning contributor of news-feature and feature articles, profiles, arts reviews and previews to local, regional, and national publications. Trainin Blank also does grant writing and book edit-ing. She has authored several plays and Her first book,* What to Do about Mama: A Guide to Caring for Aging Family Members, *was published in 2013. Her second book, a biography of Mary Sachs, is due for publication in 2015. Trainin Blank graduated from Barnard College (Columbia University). She is a native New Yorker, and lives with her professor husband in Silver Spring, Md. They have two grown children and a cat.*

# THE MAN ON MY SHOULDER
## Michelle Matthews

T he pain was fleeting. I had taken enough pain killers that I
didn't feel the sting. I didn't want to feel anymore. That was
the point. I cried, then sobbed and shook with violent tremors that
only come from the release of a lifelong pain. I didn't want to die
but I didn't want to live. I cried because I was tired. I was so tired
of dragging the one foot behind me that was deeply rooted six feet
underground.

The water burned my skin around the scratches I had inflict-
ed earlier. As I soaked, I stared at the blade resting at my side.
But the cutting was done. I was lying in a tub filled with warm water, water that hadn't quite warmed the cool porcelain. It was hot
enough to burn my skin, though, especially around the gashes.
I soaked and I stared at the blade resting beside me on the tub
edge.

Going back as far as I can remember, I was always a little off. I was a loner content to live in the shadows of my family. I would reside in the dark corners with a good book, escaping into a different world and a different life, a life where I was normal.

The first time I ever had an anxiety attack I was around eight years old. I didn't know then what it was and neither did my family. All I remember is that it was cold outside (cold weather and the change of seasons are triggers for me), and I felt like the dirt of the city was crawling all over me. It was swirling around and was going to engulf me. It was coming out of my skin, out of every pore. It made me itch and I scratched myself until my skin was raw and bleeding. After that incident, anything that was dirty set me off. I began seeing dirt that wasn't there. School was miserable—I would sit and look in the corners all day, staring at the dirt. I couldn't use the restrooms, not just because there were bullies who made my life miserable, but because it was so dirty in there. I could never get clean.

Living in my home with these phobias was not a pleasant experience. I was constantly ridiculed and made the butt of every joke. I learned to turn off my emotions and to not show I cared about what people said, but it hurt.

Even my family didn't seem to care if they hurt me. Instead of trying to help me, they found ways to set off a reaction. They made gagging sounds like they were going to throw up because they knew I had a phobia of it, which would set off a rush of adrenaline and send me into a fight or flight response. They thought it was hilarious; I thought it was cruel. I never did understand why people who were supposed to love me were so mean to me. Looking back now I realize what I suffered in my home would be considered emotional abuse.

Depression hit me hard once I entered my teens. My self-esteem was in the toilet, and whenever I looked in the mirror I was disgusted. I wanted to be pretty like the other girls in school and I was not. It was then I started cutting and scratching myself. My family's response to this behavior was, "Why would you do something to make yourself look uglier?" That's what I was told, word for word. It has stuck with me ever since. Where other people saw beauty, I saw ugliness. Depression tells lies to you; it's the bad angel on your shoulder whispering in your ear. This was the first lie depression told me, and it would not be the last.

The college years were my saving grace. The friends I made there were the counselors I never knew I needed. I had the best years of my life in college. It wasn't because I was in love, I wasn't. It wasn't because I had lots of money, I was a broke student eating ramen noodles and whatever was in the cafeteria. But I was happy because I was around people who knew I had emotional issues and they still loved me for me. They still invited me out, sometimes kicking and screaming because they knew once I got over my phobia, I would have a good time. They never expected or asked me to change. Complete acceptance can be a powerful drug to someone who has never been accepted. I've been chasing that dragon ever since.

During my college years I also found a diagnosis. A diagnosis meant I had something more to check off when I went to the doctor's office: seasonal affective disorder, depression, obsessive-compulsive disorder, and anxiety. The fantastic four! I'm a lucky girl.

In college I started medication that promised to make me normal. For the first time I saw the world through an even-keeled spy glass and the world was *boring*. There were no highs, but there also weren't any lows. For two years I felt like I experienced no emotions. Because I wanted to feel again, I went off my medication, preferring natural remedies that don't always work but were better than nothing at all.

I went through a series of bad relationships that reinforced my ever-decreasing sense of self, until eventually I married because I was afraid I was so hideous I would always be alone. I had children and discovered that being pregnant was a natural cure for me. I was emotional but I wasn't depressed. I felt the healthiest I have ever felt in my life. If it were up to me I would be perpetually pregnant, but even that option was taken away. When I had my twins, the surgeon missed a tear on my uterus. I hemorrhaged and flat-lined in the recovery room, and they had to do an emergency hysterectomy to save my life. I was thirty and in menopause.

The worst thing about trying to live with depression is how other people treat you. People I've known have yelled at me and told me that I'm "selfish," to "just get over yourself" and asked me questions like, "What do you have to be depressed about?"

If it were up to me, I wouldn't be this way. I wouldn't choose depression. I've always wanted to live a normal life like the ones depicted on TV. I always wanted the fairytale. Instead, I live an existence that I refuse to accept because I still want a fairytale that isn't attainable for someone like me. I still believe the lies that depression tells me because it's easier to say yes to the little man on my shoulder than to fight him. Fighting him is a losing battle. It's easier to believe that I'm unlovable because one more heartache might be the final straw that sends me over the edge to the place where I don't come back.

This is all true except for my children. My children are my life vests. The three of them keep me afloat more than they know. The promise of seeing what they will become is what keeps me wanting to greet the next day.

But my fear is that, one day, even they will not be enough. That fear weighs me down every September when I know my worst season starts. The days get shorter and the monster that sits at my doorstep all summer grows. Come Thanksgiving he will feast on me, tearing my life to shreds and making the people I love hate me. He will push me away from everything I love and care about and I will be powerless to stop it. All I can do is wait and pray that this won't be the year that he becomes too much to carry.

Depression makes it hard for me to have relationships. The man on my shoulder always whispers his lies and I believe him. He's the one constant in my life, always with me. He pulls me away from my friends and family, forever keeping me at arm's length from my loved ones. Depression fogs my brain and eats away at my memories. He won't be happy until I'm completely alone.

Last winter was the roughest one I have ever known. The depression seems to be getting worse as I get older, harder for me to control. In my younger days, I was just a little down; now I have days when the thought of having to live another day is paralyzing. I cry often. I sob and shake with violent tremors that should be cathartic. Only it's never enough. I don't want to die; I don't want to live. I cry because I am tired, tired of dragging one foot behind me that is deeply rooted six feet underground.

⇒⋮ ⋮⇐

But the cutting was done. I was lying in a tub filled with warm water, water that hadn't quite warmed the cool porcelain. It was hot enough to burn my skin, though, especially around the gashes. I soaked and I stared at the blade resting beside me on the tub edge.

I heard him call my name from downstairs—he was home from work and I had waited for him. I didn't want the children to see me like this. I ran the blade across my skin several times before putting it away, just as he opened the door to ask me what I was doing taking a bath in the middle of the day. I would make up some excuse like cramps. In the end, I didn't want him to see me like this.

*Michelle is a graduate of the George Washington University with a B.A. in Criminology and her love of Forensics has managed to seep into quite a few of her flash fiction pieces. A self-professed movie and TV snob, she also has an encyclopedic knowledge of all things musical. Her blog,* Scattered Wrecks, *showcases her short stories, social commentary and unsolicited advice. Her writing has been on BlogHer and Mamapedia. Michelle lives in Northern Virginia with her family.*

# DRIVING CRAZY

## Jenn Rian

W hen I say that I'm a stay at home mom, I mean it. I literally stay at home because I don't have a driver's license. Anxiety is super fun … or not. One of the ways anxiety has proved to be the most paralyzing for me is while driving a car. What began as mere nervousness in my teens has grown into delusional paranoia during adulthood. The tragically ironic part is that the *desire* to be able to drive is much stronger now than it ever was in my teens, yet so far I've been unable to conquer my fear. Those who don't understand anxiety would tell me to just get over it and face my fear head on. Hahaha hahaha hahaha, um, *no*.

I can ride in a car as a passenger with nary a worry. Once I'm behind the wheel my entire perspective changes and there is death and destruction around every corner. My driving skills are fine; I am an extremely cautious driver, to endearing "little old lady" proportions. The problem is I have such a fear of the unknown that I have no faith in how I might react in unpredictable circumstances. Before I even start the car I've already frothed myself up into a paranoid tizzy with a plethora of "what ifs." What if I don't notice important street signs such as a change in the speed limit or "Turn now lest ye fall into a pit of sewage in 5 miles!" What if the sun is so bright that it scorches my corneas and I'm unable to see to drive while I'm clawing at my face screaming, "My eyes! Dear God, my big beautiful eyes!" What if I drive too slowly and I make the driver behind me so angry that they get out of their car at the red light and yell at me? What if I'm so afraid of making the surrounding drivers impatient that I drive too fast and make the car tip to the side on two wheels when I'm turning a corner? What if I'm too close to the parked cars and I scrape against one, locking our side mirrors in an accidental yet Herculean embrace, dragging the other car along with me so that it smashes everything in front of it? What if I don't make a turn wide enough or I drive down the wrong side of the road which is inevitably crowded with semi-trailer trucks that now have to avoid colliding with me by making impossibly nimble maneuvers meant only for the smallest of vehicles? It's like living inside of Frogger except I'm both the frog and the car. Surely I will inadvertently annihilate entire families of innocent woodland creatures whilst being forced off of the road by a combination of road-ragers, random patches of ice, run-away barrels, hurricanes, and spontaneous herds of cattle. Game over. Womp-womp-womp.

It was fourteen years after receiving my first driver's permit when I finally attempted the driving portion of the test for the first and only time. I was in the first trimester of pregnancy with my second child and my husband had decided that it was time for me to get my license. He appealed to my logic; if I could get my license, I never actually had to drive again if I didn't want to. In a well-meaning, though misguided attempt at propelling me toward success, he scheduled an appointment for the driver's test without consulting me first. Surprise! Because nothing motivates someone with anxiety more than the paralyzing fear of being ill-prepared combined with the extraordinary pressure of a looming deadline. Perfect.

The driving instructors at our local DMV were mean and notorious for failing nearly everyone on their first test. Because we're sneaky opportunists we made the appointment at a different DMV where the instructors were rumored to be slightly more accommodating. I was unfamiliar with the area and extremely anxious about where I'd have to drive during the road test so we went to the DMV to practice, accompanied by my younger cousin who had recently passed his driver's test at the same location. From the DMV parking lot my cousin instructed me to make a left then make another left at the intersection and make a third left back around the median strip. It seemed simple—that is, until during one of our trips around when my husband suddenly shrieked as though we would all surely die, which startled me and I panicked. I hopped the median strip and flew diagonally past a lane of traffic into a nearby parking lot. I ripped the keys from the ignition and threw them directly at my husband's genitals without even hitting the breaks or turning off the car. Then I buried my head in my hands and burst into tears as the car rolled to a stop. Neither my husband nor I can remember why he had cried out, though I do recall at the time being quite adamant that his reasoning was completely exaggerated and unfounded.

Despite our near death experience, we figured that my driving skills were good enough as long as no one was hollering at me as though we were about to meet Jesus. Considering that driving with my husband makes me nervous because he spontaneously squawks at me like a church lady that just got Bingo, I went to the DMV while it was closed to practice parallel parking with my mother. If you don't pass the parallel parking portion of the test you don't even get the opportunity to attempt the road test. I practiced for hours and I did fine. No one screamed at me, I didn't dangerously cross lanes of traffic, and I wasn't compelled to lob my keys or any other inanimate object at my mother's external reproductive organs.

The evening before my driver's test I practiced parallel parking at home. There was a space between my mother's car and her neighbor's car. I can do this. I can do this. I ... *can't* do this. I tried three times and failed three times. I noticed the neighbor peering wide-eyed through her window like Mrs. Kravitz. Chill, lady, I got this. And then it happened. On my last attempt at parallel parking I hit my mom's car. Well, the cars *touched*. I backed into it very slowly as though my car were giving it a deliberate and well-timed kissed. I went around the block to attempt parking one more time only to find the neighbor wearing her bathrobe and a horrified expression and frantically hurrying into her car to drive it far away to safety. Judging by the incredibly dirty looks that she hurled in my direction as she drove off, you would've thought that instead of barely touching my mother's car with my bumper I had instead just backed over a talking baby unicorn that was on the verge of granting her three wishes that included the oft forbidden option of wishing for more wishes.

Test day I was an anxious mess. I rode in the passenger's seat on the way to the DMV enduring the angel-versus-devil-like bickering of my own internal dialogue. "Jenn, you drive fine when no one is yelling at you. Yeah, but you drove *over* the median strip and then ripped the keys out of the car *while it was still moving*!" My self-inflicted quarrel was interrupted when we ran into a construction detour and the GPS kept rerouting us back to the same spot. Are you kidding me?! No, seriously ... are you freaking kidding me with this right now?! We went around in circles at least three times before we found our own alternate route, at which point we were really running late. I was obviously in the perfect head-space for operating a motor vehicle while being judged by a strange man I'd never met before.

By the time we reached the DMV I was dizzy, short of breath, my heart was racing, my palms and my upper lip were sweating. You *know* it's bad when there's upper lip sweat. Despite my mental and emotional state, the driver ahead of me had just left with the instructor and my test was quickly approaching. I waited anxiously as I watched her pass her parallel parking test and drive to the entrance of the parking lot for the road test. Then she turned right. Wait, *what*?! She turned right? Not left? Why did she turn right?! Why, why, why, and also, *why*?! I had only practiced going to the left. Newsflash, people, the right isn't the left. Do you want to know what's to the right? To the right there is a crowded, nay, *completely consumed* intersection thronged with bumper-to-bumper cars that were rushing in and out of the disorienting exits and entrances of confusing parking lots in the surrounding shopping centers. To the right there were more than four lanes of traffic, an overabundance of median strips, and a super-fluity of signs warning, "This lane only! One way! Do not enter! Hey, dummy, you're going to kill us all!" and the like. The entire location was an opportunity for my worst driving fears imagined to become a reality. Well, crap.

It was my turn and I was terrified. The instructor looked over his clipboard and then said to his colleague with a chuckle, "She came all the way from Beaver because the instructors there are so mean!" After staring at the clipboard awhile longer he said, "So, Jennifer, this is your first time taking the driving test … and you're thirty-two?" He said my age as though I was decomposing before his eyes.

"Yeah, I've had my permit for so long I keep saying they should just give me an honorary license … hahaha, haha, ha, um…" *Crickets.* I'd just been reminded how obscenely old I was, I was riddled with anxiety, hormonal from pregnancy, and my meager attempt at hu-mor had fallen flat. Awesome. But it was too late to back out, so I got in the car. Trying not to cry, I pulled ahead to attempt parallel parking. I backed up and I cut the wheel. Too soon. Much, much too soon. I knew that I couldn't fix it, so rather than prolong the torture I decide to just park that bad boy as is and call it a day. I had failed and failed marvelously … and I didn't care at all. I was just so ridiculously relieved that the ordeal was over. To this day I'm not entirely certain that I didn't subconsciously fail on purpose to avoid taking the road test.

A month after failing my driver's test, my permit expired. It's been three and a half years and I haven't attempted to renew my permit. I keep telling myself that next year is the year that I'll finally do it. I'll finally get my license.

Or maybe I'll just get a chauffeur.


*Jenn Rian is a bored and sarcastic stay-at-home-mom of two who blogs and vlogs because the voices in her head tell her to. She blogs about as often as she showers, which isn't very often. You can find her blogging at her self named site,* Jenn Rian, *where she's mildly amusing and on the site* Coolest Family on the Block *where she pretends to be a Pinterest mom.*

# A LETHAL COMBINATION
## Tammy Rutledge

I wanted to die. Not really though, I just wanted the pain to end so that I couldn't feel anything else. There was a lot going on and I had lost all ability to cope. My husband had been bedridden for eight weeks followed by months of recuperation due to a workplace accident. As a result I was caring for him, our three kids, and chauffeuring my mother long distances on the days I didn't have my own lengthy commute for work. I felt like I never had a day off or even a moment to myself. My youngest was two years old and I was exhausted. No one understood, or offered to help me, no matter how much I asked. In fact, many "friends" were dropping like flies now that I no longer had extra time for them. I felt utterly and completely alone. I felt useless. I felt hopeless. I felt worthless.

Getting out of bed every day became a huge chore. I began to wake up in a full blown rage, shaking and furious that I was still exhausted with a full day ahead of me. Ironically the rage would consume what little energy I had and I loathed myself even more for wasting such a precious commodity on anger. If I wasn't full of rage, I'd be consumed with anxiety that would twist my stomach into knots and send my thoughts racing into incoherent patterns.

At the time I didn't realize that my menstrual cycle and my medicine were exacerbating my inability to cope. I was embarrassed about the severe PMS I experienced monthly, like it was a weakness I should have been able to control. When my cycles returned two-and-a-half years after the birth of my youngest, they were erratic. It took a long time for things to fall into a predictable enough rhythm to allow for proper diagnosis and treatment.

Once, after I'd started on medication for my year-round allergies, I had a random fight with my husband and I sat crying on my bed. While crying, I spotted a hunting knife he'd recently acquired sitting on the bedside. I picked it up and held it against my arm, dragging the cool blade over my skin while imagining an end to all my pain. All I would have to do is turn my arm over and push on the blade. Suddenly my skin split open under the blade, spilling small drops of warm blood. I hadn't meant to cut myself; the blade was sharper than I'd anticipated, but it felt unexpectedly good. Lightly I dragged the knife over my arm again and again, feeling the pain of each slice and relishing a weird, physical release of my mental anguish. I hadn't planned it, but my mental illness had escalated into self-harm.

When my husband saw the cuts on my arm he went ballistic. I cried and cried, ashamed of what I had done. I prayed that the cuts wouldn't leave scars, and over time they've become barely noticeable. His yelling about them though, while understandable, made me feel worse. However, it had the desired effect of stopping me from doing it again, even though the temptation held me for a while.

I wanted to reach for the knife, but instead started researching my symptoms on the Internet. I don't know what inspired me to explore the possible reactions to my medication, but in doing so I learned that my suicidal thoughts and self-harming actions could be a reaction to the medicine. I immediately stopped taking it. Although the medicine had been prescribed by my family doctor, I brought it to my psychiatrist's attention at our next appointment and he confirmed that stopping it was the right thing to do. Luckily I'd been seeing him regularly for years since suffering postpartum depression and he knew this behavior wasn't typical of me.

Fortunately my mother got her driver's license so that I could reclaim fifteen hours a week for myself, and slowly my husband recovered enough to participate in family life again. While I was no longer thinking about seeking relief in physical pain, I still wasn't me. I was still riddled with anxiety, spending sleepless nights tossing and turning, telling myself I didn't deserve anything good in this world. Anything and nothing could make me cry; I could easily work myself into tears with my own thoughts. More than once I stood at my station at work with my hair hiding my face while tears streamed silently down. I was a mess.

I started taking flax seed oil after a friend advised me it would do wonders for my hair, which has always been on the thin side. While it did *nothing* for my hair, all of a sudden I found myself with a regular menstrual cycle for the first time in my life and could confirm that my mental health issues happened during the last two weeks of my cycle. The pattern was clear and I began to learn about premenstrual dysphoric disorder (PMDD). After seeing my doctor I was prescribed an anti-depressant and I also started writing. Both have been instrumental to the well-being of my mental health. I also learned to be cautious with medications, as my mental illness can interact with even the most innocuous of drugs, including alcohol.

Shortly after I was diagnosed I wrote this poem and published it on my blog:

*Through this lens of PMDD*
*Anxiety and hopelessness are staring at me.*

*I want them to die a sudden death, leave me to finally feel peace in my breath.*
*They whisper in my ears that nothing is right. They say give up, go away, don't bother to fight.*
*They tell me bold wretched lies, and my heart breaks in pieces as I try not to cry.*
*Through this lens of PMDD*
*A doctor handed Prozac to me.*
*He said there's no shame in taking meds, a lot of people have demons inside their heads.*
*I'm taking the pills and I wait to see, if they'll have a lasting effect on me.*
*I'm taking the pills as I wait for my cycle to end*
*So I can wait two more weeks to go through this again.*

PMDD has probably caused me to ruin more than one friendship and I will forever be sorry for each and every hormonal outburst I've unleashed on anyone. Living with mental illness isn't easy, but I've learned that it's easier with help, and easier when I'm honest with others and myself. I've also learned that no matter what I'm going through, there is someone else out there going through the same thing, and I'm never really as alone as I feel.

*Tammy Rutledge is a Mother to 3 boys and a boat load of dogs. She earned a degree in Psychology with a minor in Sociology after starting her beautiful family. In her rare spare moments she's finding her voice on her blog,* Daze by Crazy, *is happily exploring the blogosphere and all the wonderful things it has to offer.*

# IN THE AFTERMATH OF LOSS
## Kathryn Leehane

I have dealt with depression my entire adult life. For the most part, I can manage it on my own. I recognize the signs, feeling in a very physical way the oppressive, sinking sensation that comes over me. It weighs down my body and makes me heavy … weary … tired. I'm drowning in a slow-moving eddy; the spinning paralyzes me and makes my vision fuzzy. People talk, but I don't hear them. I can't concentrate on what they are saying or what I am doing. My life is happening around me, but I'm surrounded by a glass wall that prevents me from participating.

Most times, I can identify when I need to stop the spinning and focus on myself. I know when to get fresh air and more exercise. I know when to head over to my Grandma's house (she's my unlicensed therapist). I know when to do the things my body needs me to do in order to help combat the fucked-up chemistry in my brain. I am very lucky that way.

Other times, when my depression is more intense, it becomes too much for me to handle on my own and I turn to a professional. These are the times when I withdraw from my family and friends. When I can't answer the phone. When I stay in bed all day. When I don't have the will to shower or even change clothes. It's at these moments that I know I need to reach out for professional help. And I do. It might take me a while, but I do.

I can live with my depression. I've become comfortable with it, and it's part of who I am. I know how fortunate I am to be able to recognize what is happening to me and how to address it. I know there are others who suffer from depression much worse than I do. I know, on a deeply personal level.

⟞⋇⟝

I hadn't seen my brother in over fifteen years. He had disengaged from the family and cut off all contact. We knew he was an alcoholic. We knew he needed help. But he was never able to ask for it and never able to let us in. Eventually, his mental illness overcame him, and he ended his life.

The business of death is sad and chaotic, and the suicide of a loved one brings with it a unique set of emotions. Because of my history, I knew I was at risk for a major depression spiral. I knew I needed to keep close tabs on myself during this emotional family crisis. I relied on my friend Nicole to help keep me in check. We'd talk and text often. She'd help me to gauge my state of mind. She was there for me when I most needed her, like when I talked with medical examiners about my brother's cause of death and how long the body had remained undiscovered.

When I interviewed funeral homes and determined what weight of body bag would be required given the advanced state of decomposition.

When I brought my parents (separately—they are divorced) to the notary to sign the cremation authorization forms.

When I wrote my brother's obituaries and submitted them to the newspapers—one in our hometown and one in the city in which he had lived alongside the friends and co-workers I never knew.

When I flew to another state to clean out his apartment, the apartment I had never been to and never seen him in.

When I disposed of all of his worldly possessions.

When I cleaned the closet where he hung himself, removing the shorn tie from the closet rod with my own two hands.

And when I prayed the "Our Father" in his bedroom before leaving that apartment for the last time.

Nicole helped me keep myself in check while I was busy being strong for my parents, who shouldn't have had to deal with the loss of their child. She helped me be strong for my other siblings, who were overcome by their own grief. She helped me be strong for my brother, whom I couldn't save.

I was so busy being strong that I didn't notice the anxiety symptoms sneaking up on me. These uninvited guests crept quietly into my life one by one—so quietly that I didn't even notice their arrival until they'd already launched their simultaneous attack.

First came the rapid heartbeat. I wrote that off as too much caffeine. I needed coffee to help me power through the day, but maybe I had had too much?

Then came the tightening in my chest. The clamp around my ribcage. My body was so tense; I needed to relax. I needed to take deep breaths.

Then came the difficulties breathing. My short, staccato breaths would take over my entire body, pinning me in place and depriving me of sufficient oxygen. I brushed them off as grief. I tossed the signs aside as I choked back my tears and kept working through the business of death.

Then came the nightmares. I had visions of my dead brother standing at the edge of my bed. Never talking. Just watching. Just waiting for me to help him.

Then came the sleepless nights. Too afraid to dream, I would lay awake for hours. I couldn't face the visions; I couldn't face my guilt.

Then came the hair loss. Clumps of hair would fall out in the shower. Strands would cling to my fingers each time I ran my hands across my head. "Damn, I really need more sleep," I would tell myself.

Somehow I functioned fine in my daily routine. I brought the kids to their activities. I took care of the dogs, the house, and the family. All of these activities kept me focused in a different direction. They kept me distracted from my anxiety's mounting assault.

Until they weren't there to distract me anymore.

One weekend, a few weeks after the memorial service and after I had closed out most of my brother's affairs, my husband took the kids to visit a friend out of town. I couldn't go because there was too much to do at home. And, quite frankly, I needed to not be strong for other people for a while. I needed to be alone and attend to myself.

I was going through my memory box, searching desperately for mementos from my brother. Looking for anything—photographs, drawings, letters. All I found was a short letter that he had written to me in college. It was a simple note introducing some sort of article that he had clipped out of the newspaper. The article was not there, but I clung to that note.

First my heart started racing and then my chest tightened. I tried to breathe through it. I closed my eyes and willed myself to breathe through it. When I opened my eyes, I felt a little better, so I pushed on. I found an old journal of mine from high school and thumbed through it. I was looking for anything I might have written about my brother. Anything at all.

That's when I read it. A journal entry, written in my own hand, describing my desire to end my life. My own words declaring my intention to hang myself in my closet. Just as my brother had done.

Suddenly everything—all of those silent enemies who had been so stealthy for so long—pounced on me all at once. Overwhelming me. Taking full control of my body. Seizing all of my senses.

I couldn't breathe. My ribcage squeezed my lungs and chest, they burned inside of me. My vision went black. My heart raced and I reached out for something to steady me. My arms flailed. I couldn't find my ground. I couldn't find a compass. My brain swirled like a tornado. It was spinning out of control. Nothing had prepared me for this. Time seemed suspended. My gut constricted. I thought I was going to die. There was no oxygen. Nothing to help me breathe. I. Could. Not. Breathe.

All I could see was his closet. The shorn tie on the rod. The clothes piled on the floor. The fluids that had fallen onto those clothes when the coroner had moved the body. The bugs that had swarmed my face while I cleaned. The mess. Oh, the mess. That tiny room was the closest I had been to my brother in over a decade, and it was all death. All soiled clothes and death.

And that tie. My brain seized upon that tie.

Then, suddenly, the panic released me. I collapsed in a heap on the floor. I wailed. I sobbed. I completely lost it—ugly, loud crying. My heart was still racing, but at least I could breathe. At least the vice on my chest had released. Cold and shivering (had I been sweating?), I picked myself up off the floor and crawled to my bed. I slept for hours.

That was the first anxiety attack. But it was far from the last. It seems that once the mental combatants joined together, they didn't want to part. They started coming fast and furious, at surprising (and not so surprising) moments: praying the "Our Father" at school drop-off, driving away from my kids' school, hearing certain songs, shopping for cleaning supplies, lying awake in my bed at night.

I knew I needed help. Professional help. But I didn't know how to ask. I couldn't discuss it with my husband or Nicole without the symptoms stirring inside of me. Thankfully, it only took a few weeks and the quiet of a morning alone to gather the courage to make the phone call and get myself to therapy.

I'm not going to lie. It took a while to start talking freely about my brother's suicide, even though my therapist diagnosed me with post-traumatic stress disorder right away. We spent many weeks discussing my brother, my guilt, the closet, that tie.

It has not been an easy road, but I'm glad I took it. I'm done with therapy, for now. The anxiety attacks haven't disappeared completely, but they have decreased in their frequency and intensity. I know most of my triggers, and can sense the attacks approaching. I can usually manage them by taking a walk, reducing my caffeine intake, or slowing down and breathing.

So I live with both anxiety and depression now, and I struggle on a daily basis. Still, I know I am fortunate. There are those who suffer far worse. Those who lose the battle. Part of my self-prescribed therapy is writing. So I write. I write to share my brother's story, to keep a part of him alive with me. I write to laugh and to make others laugh. I write to connect with people. And I write to survive.

*Kathryn Leehane is a writer and humorist living in the San Francisco Bay Area with her husband and two children. Along with inhaling books, bacon and Pinot Noir, she writes the humor blog,* Foxy Wine Pocket, *where she shares twisted (and only sometimes exaggerated and inappropriate) stories about her life as a mother, wife, friend and wine-drinker in suburbia. She is a contributing author to several anthologies and is at work on her first book--a memoir about loss and survival. Her essays have also been featured on* BLUNTmoms, The Huffington Post, Mamapedia, Megsanity, Scary Mommy, *and more.*

# CAN I GET AN AMEN?
## Linda Roy

Catholic school. Need I say more? I'm a recovering Catholic, so suffice it to say it's taken me years, some therapy, and a mental block to get over the human drama of eight grueling years of plaid-laden anxiety.

In Catholic school, mass figures into the equation a few times a week. That's roughly three hours spent sitting next to classmates and friends, desperately trying not to communicate while under the watchful hawk eye of Sister Mary Smackme, who was always poised to haul off and administer a surrender-to-Jesus moment of reckoning without notice.

With a short attention span and heavy on irreverence, I had little patience for the sit, stand, kneel, repetition of the mass ritual. The only way I was going to survive such drudgery was to be part of the show, and since I played guitar, joining the school folk group was the best plan. Rehearsals got me out of class, and I was on the holy stage in front of a captive audience, busting out killer renditions of "I Will Raise Him Up (On the Last Day)" like I was playing The Concert for Bangladesh, except this was The Concert For Jesus, and the only thing that was likely to make its way to India was my lunch money by way of a UNICEF donation box.

Catholic school was like a paramilitary organization. Whenever a classroom full of kids went anywhere, they were lined up from shortest to tallest like a spiritual von Trapp Family. Usually the shortest person in the class, I was always first in line. Being the shortest definitely sucked, but the Bible does say, "the last shall be first," so I guess that was God's way of giving me a little heads up above the competition. And at least in terms of the lunch line, it was a win, especially on pizza day.

This is how we were shepherded through the halls of Our Lady of Perpetual Guilt into the dimly lit church for mass. Upon our arrival the line order was reversed, as if we were backing a U-Haul into God's parking space. Because God is all-merciful, but His henchmen are not, Sister Mary Smackme crowded us into a tiny railed-off space on one side of the altar. Rows of prayer candles lined the wall behind us as the Virgin Mary hovered overhead. To our right the pastor, Father Canon, worked the stage, pacing back and forth during his sermon like a hopeful for best in show at the American Kennel Club Championship. Our immediate left held a small bowl of holy water perched precariously inside a metal ring bolted to the wall.

There I was, in all my glory, front and not quite center with my guitar, sharing the stage with the Almighty, a wordy spastic priest, and the other members of my musical kumbaya kinship. With very little room between myself and a filled-to-the-brim cup of holy water, I was forced to angle the neck of my guitar slightly upward to keep my distance.

It was Lent season, which meant Passion of the Christ time, so a copious amount of sit, stand, kneel action was definitely in the cards. But for those of us in the folk group, it just meant lots of standing. It sort of made me wish I'd given up standing for Lent. Literally, for the love of God, couldn't we just have sat down? But as these things go, the more you suffer, the more pious you are. Besides, who wants to be the asshole who complains during the Passion of the Christ? "I can't *stand* for an hour and a half!"

Over the course of ninety minutes we amused ourselves during psalms, open letters to the Ephesians or whoever, and a run-on sermon. My fidgeting reached epic levels. Hell, we all fidgeted. One kid chewed on his tie. Another threw spit-balls. Spit balls! I chewed on my guitar pick and stared at my Buster Brown saddle shoes.

That's when I noticed my shoelace was untied. Even then I was a tad obsessive-compulsive; I became completely fixated with worry over the errant shoelace. What if I tripped over it on my way to Communion, falling flat on my face, ending up with my plaid pleated skirt up around my neck, and my underwear in full view of a congregation full of prepubescent rubberneckers?

So up there on the altar, somewhere during the collective monotone recitation of the Apostles' Creed, I was plotting my next move.

"I believe in the Father Almighty, Maker of heaven and earth..."

Hmm, if I just bend down slowly, crouch down, balancing the guitar...

"...of all that is seen and unseen..."

...I can tie the shoe really quick, get back up, and hopefully no one will notice.

"...and to the Republic, for which it stands..."

Wait. What?

Now! I have to do it *now!*

Everyone was in a trance-like stupor, blathering by rote. I slowly bent down, carefully balancing the neck of the guitar on one knee, while balancing my weight on the other knee. Ever so discreetly, I tied the lace. All was right again in my anxiety-riddled world.

Just then, the room fell silent. I realized that the prayer was over and the priest was doing something important. All eyes were pointed in my direction. Not wanting to look like the doofus on the floor

tying a shoelace while balancing a guitar, I shot up to a standing position and as I did, the neck of my guitar hit the bottom of the holy
water cup! The cup catapulted, seemingly in slow motion up over our
heads, giving us all a symbolic baptismal soaking.

My performance did not go over well with Father Canon or Sister
Mary Smackme, both of whom were staring an imaginary laser beam-
like hole through my forehead. The whole place went dead silent and
all attention was on little sacrilegious me. Sister Mary Smackme just
glared as I managed to eke out a weak, "Forgive me, I know not what
I've done…?"

And then, like a gift from heaven, Father Canon moved on to the
next holy order of business. Hallelujah! I was off the hook. That is until we got back in the classroom, where the Lenten passion continued
in a more personal manner for me via Sister Mary Smackme's well
worn wooden paddle.

Corporal blows as a result of some misplaced H2O? I think even
Impassioned Jesus would've found that insufferable, too.

Can I get an Amen?


*Linda Roy is a writer and musician living in New Jersey with her husband
and two boys. Her blog* <u>elleroy was here</u> *is a mix of humor and music she refers
to as "funny with a soundtrack". She was named a 2014 BlogHer Voice of
the Year for humor and has co-authored several anthologies. She is a regular
contributor at* The Huffington Post *and* Humor Outcasts *and her work
has been featured at Scary Mommy,* In the Powder Room, Erma Bombeck
Writers' Workshop, BlogHer, Mamapedia, BonBon Break, Midlife
Boulevard, Aiming Low, *and* The Weeklings.

# I WASN'T EXPECTING THIS

## Lynn L. Shattuck

It's April Fool's Day when the first wave of nausea hits. My two-year-old son's preschool is closed due to a freakishly late snowstorm. Max stands at the front windows, his round face tilted up, watching giant clumps of snow fall from the sky. As I'm mentally rearranging my day to accommodate the unexpected, something like seasickness hits me, then fades. A few minutes later, I feel another roll of queasiness.

I open my laptop and turn on an Elmo video for my son. "Here you go. Mama will be right back, okay?" I say, before darting up to the second floor bathroom.

"O-tay," Max chirps, his eyes already focused on the video.

I grab a leftover pregnancy test from before Max was born, and I quickly pee on it. A pink plus sign spreads across the test.

"Ohmygod," I whisper.

"Mama!" Max hollers from downstairs.

"Coming!" I yell.

Ohmygod.

I tell my husband Scott that night, as he is wiping stray snowflakes off his collar.

"Are you serious?" he asks. He's wide-eyed but smiling.

"I guess I miscalculated when I was ovulating," I admit. We stand in the kitchen, while Max stomps around the living room.

"Are you happy?" Scott asks.

"I don't know," I say. "I guess."

And for a few days, I am. My husband and I had hit a very rough patch a few months earlier, and this feels like a sign of hope for us. A new start.

From another perspective, I just finally weaned my son after twenty-six months. I had recently stopped going to the postpartum depression group I'd attended since two weeks after his birth. I was thinking of starting writing again, or maybe looking for a part-time job.

My life was just starting to feel like my own again.

⋘ ⋙

A week later, I am decidedly *not* happy. The hormonal chaos from pregnancy and weaning has hit hard. My son's night waking still shatters my sleep. The exhaustion I've felt for the last two years intensifies from the work my body is doing to grow another person. I feel helpless to all this change—against my will, cells are dividing, hormones hurtling through my blood, making me weepy and nauseous.

I've had several bouts with depression, the most recent being of the postpartum variety after Max's birth. I didn't realize it could strike *during* a pregnancy. But this is how depression moves; it sweeps in whether you're expecting it or not, lowering its net around you.

The nausea intensifies. The thought of food disgusts me, despite the fact that I feel weak. One night I come downstairs to a terrible stench. "What in the world are you doing?" I ask my husband, covering my mouth.

"I'm cooking broccoli," he answers.

"It smells like death," I say, gagging. Usually, I like broccoli.

The fierce undertow of exhaustion and nausea suck me down. When I stand up, little black spots threaten my vision.

And then there's my son. My spirited, strong-willed two-year-old. I let him watch hours of Elmo every day while I stare off into the distance, feeling like a terrible mother. I try to bribe him into naps so I can lie down myself. He usually doesn't take the bait. I burst into tears when he does two-year-old things, like refuse to get in his car seat.

But mornings are the worst.

I open my eyes and depression greets me, sallow and sure. Another day of exhaustion and dry heaving and dizziness awaits me. Another day encased in the miserable fog I can't push away. And beyond today, when I can squint beyond it, I see months upon months of fatigue, puking, and then, after all of that, another baby. Even less sleep. Two kids in diapers. Zero time to myself. And probably another round with postpartum depression.

"I can't do this," I say to my husband in the morning.

"You can," he says.

I stare at the white ceiling above our bed and say, "I feel like I can't and I need you to be okay with that." He hugs me and tries to meet me where I am, but if you have ever experienced depression, you know that people can't really meet you where you are. It is a murky, shrouded place that spouts a constant stream of distorted thoughts. You look like yourself, but behind your eyes is the worst version of you, lost and dark.

"Okay," he says.

I give my son baths and crouch next to the tub writing in my journal, my tears smudging the ink. I pray for a miscarriage. I'd always planned on having two children, but not like this. Not if it means losing myself just as I was finally coming up for air, surfacing.

When I drive past the nearby Planned Parenthood, I stare at the building and wonder if I'll be walking through those doors in the next week.

I tell my therapist about my doubts. "Thirty-seven-year-old married people don't get abortions," I say.

"They do. They absolutely do. Far more often than you would think," she says with conviction. She has sat in her chair talking with clients for many, many years, and I believe her. I began seeing her when postpartum depression hit me right after my son was born. She knows about the struggles in my marriage and the difficulty I've had adjusting to becoming a parent. I have no doubt that she wants the best for me.

On the long days with my son, when he whines and cries and I feel like a zombie in my sick, drained body, each minute feels unbearable. I am buffered from hope, as I have been each of the times I've experienced depression.

Getting an abortion feels like the only escape. The only exit from this maze of hormones.

"I can't do this," I say to my husband again, on another morning.

He just looks at me. He reaches for my hand.

And yet. I stare at my son's face.

Before having Max, I could've had an abortion. I didn't, but I could have, if the circumstances had called for it. But after having a child, it's not so easy to disassociate. Not when I can see what waits at the end of this swarm of cells: a small, breathing creature who has my eyes and my strong will. My husband's mouth and easy disposition.

One day when I drive by Planned Parenthood, I think, *But what if this is my little girl?* Having always imagined myself the mother of a daughter, I let my fingertips touch my belly. I contemplate that I'm housing the small seed of a baby instead of just a detonating hormone bomb.

I find out that one of my best mom friends, the one I sip coffee with while we try to peel away from our two-year-olds, is pregnant, too. I grasp onto these slivers like life jackets, and for small moments, I feel relief.

I make some phone calls to my midwife. I get a prescription to take the edges off my nausea, and a higher dose of the antidepressants I already take.

Within days, the fog lifts, as strangely as it descended. I don't feel happy about my pregnancy; I feel something more like resignation, which slowly blooms into acceptance. Happiness will come later, when she—yes, it is a she—is in my arms. When she falls asleep on my shoulder, a smudge of sun streaking her face. When she finally, at nine weeks, smiles, and then never stops.

I make a plan in case the depression returns after she is born. My parents will help out with Max. I see a psychiatrist, and we have a medication plan. I know about the postpartum support group, and I get the name of a postpartum doula to have on hand.

I survive.

We survive.

When she is born, the midwife places her on my chest. "Is she still a girl?" I ask. She is tiny and wet and light in my arms. She has pale skin and blue eyes. For a long moment, we take each other in. Within minutes, she squirms toward my nipples, turned near-black by hormones. She drinks, somehow knowing that I am hers, even if at first, all those months ago, I wasn't sure that she was mine.


*Lynn Shattuck grew up in an Alaskan rainforest and now live in the 'burbs of Maine. Her favorite stories have to do with truth-telling, imperfection, spirit, parenting, and grief. Lynn blogs at* <u>The Light Will Find You</u>, <u>Mom.me</u>, *and* <u>The Elephant Journal</u>. *Her work has also recently been featured in* Brain, Child *magazine and in the anthology,* Clash of the Couples.

# ON THE INSIDE

## Abby Heugel

Within the first hour of my stay in the psychiatric hospital for depression, OCD, and an exercise obsession, I had already pissed off my roommate simply because she heard me call her a weirdo on the phone. Yes, I felt bad after she started freaking out, but she was leaving the next day anyway, so as long as she didn't kill me in my sleep I figured we were okay.

In my defense, she *was* a weirdo.

From the second I arrived with my bag full of things that wouldn't go against the rules—no belts, shoelaces, drawstrings on hoodies or sweatpants, sharp objects, files to stick in baked goods— I could tell she was the kind of person who, if I were forced to interact with her on a daily basis without medication, would make me want medication.

My bag had barely touched the generic hospital bed sheets when she proceeded to tell me exactly everything that was wrong with her world, how it was somehow my fault for invading her space, that she was going to sneak in exercise between the mandatory 30-minute nurse check-ins, and that she was leaving soon so I shouldn't get too attached.

I didn't think that would be a problem, and decided to go explore the confines of the ward that would house me for an indefinite amount of time.

Now, I understand that puzzles and coloring supplies—no pencil sharpeners, of course—were available to pass the boredom, but you really shouldn't leave a 500-piece puzzle around people with OCD. Let's just say I set some sort of record for completing a puzzle in one sitting. There was a piece missing however, which haunted me for days, but puzzles were still a great way to kill time between therapy, naps, and meals.

The thing about meals in a psychiatric hospital is that when you're on the eating disorder spectrum in any way, you are lumped with the other girls/women at each meal in the cafeteria and subjected to a) tray-sitting, in which nurses sit at your table to ensure you're not "engaging in behavior" or hiding food and b) sitting at the table for an hour after each meal to ensure you're not going back to your room to purge.

It's just as glamorous as it sounds.

And while I had a hard time with the incredibly large amounts of food I was forced to eat—about three times that of a normal adult in an effort to stabilize my health—I did it because that's why I was there and I didn't want to stay any longer than I had to but also because I didn't want to piss off Nurse Ratched, as that would ensure I got the crappy desserts at every meal.

As I sat there in the cafeteria diligently eating, I was subjected to the strange rituals of some of those girls trying to hide food who threw epic tantrums and plastic sporks. They covered their meals with enough pepper and random condiments to make the food look more like a dare than a dinner. Part of it was their obsession with not actually eating and enjoying the food, and part of it was a way to regain some attention.

There was a day when Briana—a teenager on her third stay in three years—got caught slipping a cookie down her pants. A cookie. Down her pants. A coochie cookie, if you will. And she would have gotten away with it if it wasn't for the fact that her pants were hanging off her like a sheet on a two-by-four. Standing up caused the dessert to descend down her pant leg and onto the floor, at which time Mayor, a fifty-year-old manic depressive high-end attorney, came running across the room and asked if she was planning on eating it.

She was given a warning and a supplement drink. Mayor was given a look that could kill, but unfortunately (fortunately?) for him, not the cookie.

This wasn't the first time Briana caused a scene that could have qualified for an audition in *Girl, Interrupted*. The previous day they had shifted our rooms across the hall, and let's just say when you're dealing with a group of girls/women who already have issues with change, control, and routine, springing this information on them does not go over well.

While I quickly packed up and roamed down the hall like a neurotic nomad seeking the promised land, Brianna—cafeteria queen of clandestine cookie capers—took it upon herself to throw all her belongings into the hall and then throw a tantrum like a toddler who was refused a snack at the checkout counter. Despite my slightly dulled reflex time due to meds, I was still quick enough to duck when her shower sandal went flying over my head.

All in all, it was a highly entertaining performance.

Three out of four stars, my friends.

As if Brianna's hysterics weren't entertaining enough, along with sandal sling-shots we were also given the opportunity to express our feelings through both art and occupational therapy.

On one particular day that had us painting wood trinket boxes and welcome mats instead of our usual craft of trying to cut through construction paper with kid-safe scissors, Al, the eighty-five-year-old with schizophrenia, was caught smelling all the paint and glue and put on "watch;" Sarah, the suicidal thirty-year-old opera singer from New York, created a mosaic jewelry box she said she was going to keep her pot in; and Donna, a fifty-something-year-old alcoholic, sketched a self-portrait that could be sold in a gallery.

Me? I painted a welcome mat. Yes, for just $1,000 a day, you too can make a doormat to take home at the end of your stay!

What I also took home at the end of my stay was a rekindled desire to be the next Beyonce, only white and Polish with a pancake ass. One day we walked into the therapy room to find a karaoke machine. What this meant was that a group of psychiatric patients at different levels of drug-induced stupor and treatment were being asked to sing into a microphone like they were hanging out in a bar.

Let the good times roll.

At first, no one was really into it except the group leader, who valiantly tried to get us excited with the safe choice of "YMCA," appropriate considering we looked like the lost Village People.

But after a few lame attempts from others, Mayor grabbed the microphone and proceeded to bust out some "Brown Eyed Girl" that got everyone going—clapping, singing, you name it—including Al and even Briana. Pretty soon people were taking turns and everything from "Bohemian Rhapsody" to a rousing rendition of "Love Shack" from Sarah the opera queen could be heard all the way down the hall. Nurses and aids were walking by to see what was going on, and a few even stopped in and started dancing with us on the floor.

Now I can't sing, but when you're among a group of people who have seen you only at your worst, what have you got to lose?

"I Will Survive" came on and the microphone was thrust at me. Obviously having nothing better to do, I gave it a shot. You would have thought I was auditioning for *American Idol*—while wearing yoga pants, slippers, a monitor, and sporting two days of unwashed hair, much like most of the contestants in the early rounds.

I sang that song like my life depended on it, because maybe at that point, it almost did. All the stress, all the pressure, all the ups and downs of the past week—the past year—came spilling out into that song.

And while I stood there singing—watching that group of eclectic people who were so different but also alike in so many ways—I couldn't help but feel grateful. Everyone's a weirdo in their own way, and as long as we could embrace that and find the humor amidst the fog, I figured we would all be okay.

We would survive.


*Abby is a freelance writer, editor and award-winning blogger at* <u>Abby Has Issues</u>. *Her work has been featured multiple times on* The Huffington Post, Scary Mommy, Your Tango, Thought Catalog, Bustle, XO Jane, In the Powder Room *and* Erma Bombeck Writers' Workshop *among others. She has also self-published two books of her humor essays available on Amazon. When not online, she can be found eating green things from the ground and running mental marathons in yoga pants.*

# A FINE LINE

## Sarah del Rio

I was introduced to mood swings by the onset of adolescence. Luckily, I wasn't flying blind. Society had given me plenty of warning about what to expect. After all, it was 1988 when I got my first period, and back then it was still considered acceptable for people to engage in inappropriate menstrual rhetoric. Tactless PMS jokes abounded, as did "bitchy teenage girl" Hollywood stereotypes, and crass comments from men and boys everywhere along the lines of, "God, is she on the rag or what?" Given everything I'd heard in school, and everything I'd seen on *Degrassi Junior High*, I think it's safe to say I was fully prepared to be a bitchy, crybaby mess during my monthlies.

Oh, the '80s. What a fine time to be alive.

Thankfully, my pubescent mood swings turned out to be nowhere near as bad as pop culture and my junior high classmates had assured me they would be. There was definitely an "I'm going to be an insufferable crab-ass today, and you can bet I'll be drowning in the bottom of a box of Kleenex tomorrow" aspect to them—but the swings themselves didn't last very long, and they were fairly predictable. Honestly, when it came to my teenage periods, I worried way less about the mood swings and way more about the possibility that I might have to wear a sweater tied around my waist for a week.

Unfortunately, this breezy lack of concern over my mood swings did not last.

About halfway through college, my mood swings began to worsen. They went from lasting a couple of days to lasting a couple of weeks. My brief, bitchy flare-ups became long, dismal exercises in melancholy and Morrissey. Even the term "mood swing" stopped making much sense in terms of describing the problem—there was no actual swinging involved. Only a slow descent, with an extended stay at the bottom.

It became evident that my moods were no longer just hormonal in nature. They bore little resemblance to what I'd come to associate with my menstrual periods, and what's more, the timing was completely off. The fact of the matter was that these new mood swings did not demonstrate any real evidence of correlation with my cycle. They could happen any day of the month, and often did.

It was also around this time I started to develop some strange and compulsive behaviors. I would hide from the world in empty classrooms and unoccupied bathrooms. I would trail complete strangers around campus, people I obsessed over from afar, but who never even knew I existed. I would spend inordinate amounts of time carving up tables and door frames with phrases like "help me," "I'm scared," and "I hate myself."

If someone had asked me why I felt compelled to do these things, I don't think I could have ever articulated my reasons—and engaging in habits that I couldn't justify or explain was an extremely frightening concept. A combination of intense fear from my compulsions and overwhelming sadness from my mood swings was my default state of mind. Every cell in my body wanted me to find an isolated place where I could hide and wallow.

I eventually reached a point where it became a Herculean task just to leave my room and go to class. The only thing that kept me from completely succumbing to my fear and depression—and I mean the *only* thing—was the fact that I was putting myself through school, and a substantial portion of my financial aid came from academic scholarships. Skipping lectures meant failing classes, which meant losing those scholarships, which meant having to drop out of college.

So I persevered. I showed up to work. I got good grades. I socialized when I couldn't figure out any way to avoid it. I disguised my moods and compulsive behaviors as best I could, and I did a pretty decent job of faking my way through the life of a typical college student. I'm sure to most people I seemed pretty okay.

But I wasn't okay. Inside I felt disjointed, otherworldly, and sluggish. I felt like I was crawling and scraping my way through each day, kind of like that ghost chick in *The Grudge,* only with less matted hair and fewer death rattles. Everything scared me, and nothing felt right. I hated the life path I was on. I felt trapped in my relationships. My world view was dismal and overcast.

It wasn't long before it became crystal clear that I needed help.

Making that first appointment to talk to the doctor wasn't easy. I wasn't just scared—I was scared *shitless.* And can you blame me? It was the mid-90s by that point, and most Americans were still sadly undereducated about the complexities of mental illness. I know I was. I had myself completely convinced that my doctor was going to take one look at me, throw me in a psych ward, and let me descend into an undignified and irrevocable madness. I'd read *The Bell Jar.* I'd read *The Yellow Wallpaper.* I'd read *Girl, Interrupted.*

Even when I could persuade myself that my doctor wasn't going to lock me in some dusty Victorian attic and throw away the key, I was still terrified of the possibility of being medicated. The leading antidepressant of the day had been on the market less than ten years by this time, and the media had not been kind. People were constantly speculating about whether or not taking it led to violence and aggression, and there was always some new exposé linking the drug with increased suicide rates. But back then it seemed like it the solution was either this antidepressant or tranquilizers, and who wanted to spend the rest of their life on tranquilizers? The whole thing just smacked of a lose–lose situation.

And let's not forget that in those days, there was still a very real social stigma attached to the diagnosis of a mental illness or mood disorder. Back then, I would *never* have casually admitted to my depression like I do today. I know that sounds shallow, but I was twenty years old! I *was* shallow! I was petrified I'd have to spend the rest of my life dodging labels like "crazy," "emotionally fragile," or "totally incapable of getting her shit together."

Yet, in spite of all these fears and misgivings, I could not continue to live as I had been. I had to go to the doctor. I had to seek help.

So I went.

The appointment turned out to be nothing like what I'd expected. My doctor did not immediately dismiss my concerns as ridiculous or foolish. He did not heedlessly whip out the prescription pad and start scribbling out endless orders for pharmaceutical remedies. He did not panic, run out the door, and call in the padded wagons.

What he did do was talk to me.

We talked at length about my moods. We tried to pinpoint how severe they were, and how often I was having trouble with them. We brainstormed about possible triggers and what I might look into as far as healthy coping mechanisms. We discussed my sleep patterns, my diet, my energy levels, and other medications I was taking. We identified and analyzed my concerns, my fears, and my preconceived notions about mental illness.

Looking back, I'm sure that 90 percent of the questions my doctor asked me were textbook for physicians screening for depression. But it doesn't matter. That isn't what resonates in my memory. What does resonate is how my doctor managed to put my distressed twenty-year-old self at ease while assuring me that my concerns were legitimate and not uncommon, that there were courses of treatment available to me that did not involve electroshock therapy, psych wards, or a legion of Nurse Ratched wannabes, and that there were people out there who cared.

I left my doctor's office that afternoon with an official diagnosis of clinical depression. Despite that, I felt so much more confident in myself—so much more in control. That very day I began to think of myself not as a crazy person, not as a woman with a weak mental constitution, but as someone who had the misfortune to suffer from a congenital chemical imbalance.

I started a course of medicine, which to my utmost relief and delight has done an amazing job of helping me better cope with my moods for going on twenty years now. I started to seek out different and better ways of managing my disorder, while at the same time acknowledging that there would be times I would just have to ride it out. Because with this illness there will always be dark places, and for the first time in my life, I was beginning to understand and accept that.

I am almost forty now. I'm not going to lie and say it's been easy. There have been many nights when I sat fully-clothed in my empty bathtub, sobbing to the point of headache and hyperventilation. There have been desperate fugues that threw me back to my college days and the old habit of carving words of self-loathing into the doors and door frames. There have been many days when I would sit in my cubicle or at my desk, not working, just staring into the middle distance, completely devoid of emotion or interest in my own life. Not thinking of suicide, necessarily. Just not caring if I kept living.

It's a fine line.

But what I learned from my doctor so many years ago—that I was not some kind of hopeless basket case, that what I had was a physiological disorder which could be treated if not cured, that I was one of many and in no way alone—these things always helped me to get through the bad times. I know that I am fortunate in that my depression is not so crippling that I can't live a normal life.

*Sarah del Rio is a comedy writer whose award-winning humor blog <u>est. 1975</u> brings snark, levity, and perspective to the ladies of Generation X. Despite being a corporate refugee with absolutely no formal training in English, journalism, or writing of any kind, Sarah somehow manages to find work as a freelance writer and editor. Sarah contributes regularly to blog* BLUNTMoms, *has made several appearances on the* Huffington Post Best Parenting Tweets of the Week List, *and her blog won* Funniest Blog in The Indie Chicks 2014 Badass Blog Awards. *She has also been featured on* Scary Mommy, In the Powder Room, *and* The Erma Bombeck Writers' Workshop.

# SHE UNDERSTANDS CRAZY
## Leighann Adams

My scarf was snug around my neck as I walked quickly through the parking lot. Though I was certain I would be late, I hadn't left any earlier than usual, despite the fact that my appointment was half an hour earlier than it typically was.

I pulled the scarf up farther on my face and attempted to keep the wind out, tripping as I crossed the lot.

"Shit!" My boot caught on a stone and I lost my footing, sliding on the gravel.

Looking up at the row of windows I wished I could disappear instead of being on my ass on the ground, cold, on display in front of the building.

I picked myself up and hurried inside, its brick front distressed from years of weather and wear. The main walkway was newly renovated using donor money. The doors swung open automatically which was fine with me; I was sure I had broken my ankle.

But maybe I just broke my pride.

I walked the long hallway and was warmed, though I refused to take my coat off. Its heat was keeping me cozy and making me feel secure in, what I deemed, one of the worst places I had to visit every month.

The elevator rattled as it took me up to the third floor, the crazy floor, throwing itself around as though I wasn't the only one that was a little unstable. When it opened, I came face to face with a resident who muttered, "Good afternoon, ma'am," and then off he went.

*Good afternoon? What was good about it? I fell on my ass in the parking lot, froze to death walking in here, and now I have to find out if I'm still crazy. Betcha I am!*

I found a seat in the waiting room, which was jam-packed with people. Some were reading magazines circa 1974, others were tapping their feet on the floor to a non-existent beat, and another person had begun to tear paper from a book that didn't belong to her. Curling up into my coat I focused on my phone and zoned out, refusing to make eye contact or look up. These people were crazy!

Wait.

If I thought they were crazy what did they think of me, with my head jammed in my coat and my face stuffed into my phone?

Nah!

After five minutes my back began to sweat, but I refused to remove my safety. My knee was bouncing. I was anxious and ready to get my appointment over with. The room was getting smaller by the second and the other people were getting closer and closer. I was uncomfortable and didn't want to engage in small talk, which is exactly what the people in the room had started to do.

I convinced myself that I would be fine; they knew I wasn't crazy, they didn't think that about me. My knee bounced more emphatically and my eyes darted around the room. I could feel the sweat beading on my forehead and my heart beating faster. I was certain the doctor had forgotten about me.

I checked the clock on my phone and realized that it was fifteen minutes past my appointment time. I mentally prepared myself to get up to check if I was next. *Had they forgotten I was there, maybe they cancelled and didn't notify me? I shouldn't be left waiting this long, I needed out of this tiny room pronto!*

The anxiety was creeping up, forcing me to whittle away the fingernails on my left hand. I was starting on my right when my doctor came in and called my name. I leapt from my chair and bounded into her office, happy to escape the confines of the waiting room and the judgment of the people sitting there.

My doctor could see I was highly agitated. She asked how I was feeling.

"Fine, but I think you have a lot of cases out there that you need to take care of!"

And then she turned the focus back to me. She expressed her concerns over my leg bouncing, my avoiding social situations, my belief that everyone else is crazy, my anxiety attacks.

Thus began a dialogue that would last for years, where I would come to learn that I was one of the "crazy" ones. Eventually I would accept I was someone who needed to lean on professional help and it was okay.

Being in that waiting room is a huge step for a lot of people. It was for me.

We would end our sessions with my doctor asking me to look back on our previous sessions and compare before to now. How was I doing compared to those first few months? It took a lot of work, a lot of therapy, and a lot of time, but gradually the blaming, leg bouncing, and extreme anxiety began to diminish and I began to see my illness for what it was.

I can't say that I'm fixed, I can't say that I'm not a little "crazy," but I can say I've come a long way, and if it wasn't for that office (every month), that waiting room (I loathe), and that doctor (I love) I never would have made it.

*You can find Leighann at* <u>Multitasking Mumma</u> *where she writes about allergy awareness, mental health advocacy, and family hilarity. She has been featured in World Mom's Blog and on Blogher. She lives happily with her husband and daughter in Ontario Canada where she works full time while pursuing her writing career.*

# SNACK ATTACK

## Noelle Elliott

I t was late one Monday night when the school snack basket launched its attack in our kitchen. The snack basket is a bastard without a home and it always wants food. It is the school's "subtle hint" to fill the basket and return it the next day for the other children in your child's class. I have four sons and each child is required to bring a snack for the class each month. I may stink at math, but I'm confident that means the damn basket needs to be filled *all the time*. I can barely decide what food to put in my own mouth, and now I have to figure out what to feed twenty-seven other mouths?

If my children went to a normal school I could just throw in a couple of granola bars, but my kids attend a private school with very strict dietary guidelines and my husband is a teacher there. How in the world can I easily feed a classroom of kids without including gluten, dairy, sugar, nuts or for lack of a better word, *flavor*? But the school is our bread and butter, or in this case, our flax seed pita and hemp spread, so I have to go along with the rules.

I do understand the reasoning for these rules. Sugar and junk food can have an adverse effect on children, as anyone can see if they watch my kids on any given evening in our house.

So I stood in my kitchen trying to decide what to put in the hungry beast of a basket. I was tempted to purchase a box of organic mulch and pass it off as homemade trail mix as I peered into my pantry and saw a variety of cereals in various colors, a box of croutons, and a can of vegan cream of mushroom soup. The soup has been there since 2011 because it was rejected by the last food drive we had; apparently even the hungry are not that desperate. I realized I would have better luck exploring the back yard to find a suitable snack. Those acorns all over my grass were looking really appetizing at this point; once again the Snack Bastard had stumped me.

The presence of a snack basket in the average kitchen may be nothing more than a nuisance, but for someone with anxiety and obsessive-compulsive disorder, it is hell in a hand basket.

The previous week I had witnessed the glorious snack that Mama Cass brought in for all the starving kids. Mama Cass is the queen of the snack basket, and Her Hippie Hemp-ness had filled the bastard with homemade, individually wrapped, blackberry chia and lime fruit leather tied with twine. Personally, I thought the basket she brought it in sounded more appetizing than the food in the basket, but Mama Cass has her own fan club at the school and the Hemp-ness worshipers were all abuzz about her stupid fruit leather. I am sure my invitation to the fan club was lost in the mail.

There is a Mama Cass at every school. She is the mom who inadvertently makes me (and other mortal moms like me) feel inadequate.

My Mama Cass is the earthy type. On snack day she even had her hair in non-ironic pigtails. I have a solid rule to never trust a grown woman in pigtails. She wasn't wearing any make up, and it appeared that she was wearing an outfit made entirely of hemp. Generally, she has a yoga guru calm about her, which sharply contrasts with my energy signature: barista on the last hour of her shift.

Mama Cass doesn't drink coffee because her inner energy fuels her. I drink coffee because my inner energy fell asleep after my first child. Although she is a bit more granola than I would like, I must admit she is everything I had envisioned myself to be before I actually had children.

I probably focus a little bit too much on her. Did I forget to mention that my fantasy also paints her as a perfect mother? I'm entirely aware that it is a little nutty for a woman to fantasize about the home life of another woman, or at least that is what my therapist tells me. But this morning, when I was shoving my son's foot into his shoe because he has developed a sudden aversion to footwear, I thought about her. I doubt Mama Cass has a problem getting her kids to wear shoes. Perhaps it's the fact that they all wear Birkenstocks, but even if they didn't, I bet they'd happily put on their assigned footwear before climbing into their Prius and heading to school. If Mama Cass could make a hemp-woven, fruit leather culinary delight surely I could make or buy something edible to place in the bastard of a basket. After all, my bar is much lower and my kids have learned they are not living with any version of Mama Cass, but instead with a frazzled working mom just trying to make it to tomorrow.

So when I saw the Snack Bastard appear in my home this time, it was as if Mama Cass herself was challenging me not just to provide a snack, but to demonstrate my mama-cred. I silently cursed the person who put our children in the same class and did what any cookery reject does—I went to Pinterest. I had my mind set on a kiwi and grape creation that looked like a turtle. It would even tie in with the ocean theme they were studying. I was going to be a rock star! That idea quickly died when I learned I would have to cut a grape into fourths. There are twenty-seven kids in the class, which equals … 108 grape pieces? Oh, *hell* no. My turtle idea drowned.

Feeling defeated, I went to the store. After what felt like an eternity of walking up and down the natural food aisle, I decided on pre-sliced fruit knowing very well it was neither grown locally nor organic. I could have opted for the organic fruit platter, but I had spent most of my money on the Frappuccino I was drinking.

When I arrived home I arranged the fruit on a plate in the likeness of SpongeBob, which is, after all, ocean-themed. The next day my snack was a hit, even with the kids who had apparently never even watched television. Sure, I got questionable looks, because even I know pineapples don't grow in Indiana, but unlike Mama Cass, I don't have time to endlessly slice things, nor do I have the burning ambition to be a fruit tanner.

Even though the kids loved it, I still felt defeated in a competition I had created in my mind. The funny thing is that I'm not even sure this woman knows I exist. Just because she chooses an organic, natural approach to parenting and I embrace preservatives may mean her home is more Zen, but it doesn't make her children any smarter, funnier or more loved than mine.

At times my mental illness is like an obnoxious bully who cuts in line and steps in front of everyone and everything else of my life. It is my job to put it in check and send it back to its place: the back of the line.

I decided that the next time the Snack Bastard appears in my kitchen, which will probably be tomorrow, I'm not going to try to make something impossible or strive to be someone I'm not. I'm working with what I have, which means vegan mushroom soup and cereal. It's the thought that counts right?

*Noelle lives in the Midwest where she works in publicity at a university. She is a contributing writer for* Family and Sassy *magazines and has been featured on several websites including* Elephant Journal, Yahoo, Erma Bombeck *and* Tabata Times. *She is a contributing writer at* In The Powder Room. *She is the creator of the acclaimed staged production* The Mamalogues, Dramas from Real Mamas. *Noelle is the force behind the blog* Bow Chica Bow Mom, *where she writes about her lofty mission to raise the next generation of gentleman.*

# MY DARKEST DAY

## Carin Ekre Anderson

I wake each morning to the sun shining in my eyes and a song playing in my head. The song is usually a good indicator of which mood will dominate my day and what feelings I might need to be careful of. The sun either inspires me, making me grateful for the beautiful world God gave us, or it irritates me.

Clinically noted for the first time at age fifteen, and several times by other professionals, my official diagnosis is bipolar disorder. My sisters say I'm creative, stubborn, strong, generous, willful, and bitchy. My husband says I'm just fine, while others say I'm crazy.

*I* don't think I'm crazy, but I've certainly been there before. The morning inventory is one of my tricks to keep from going back. I've been checking my feelings for so long now it's habit, and how I envy people who just feel things and allow each emotion to run its own course. I have often said to people, "I don't just feel things, I *feel* things, ya dig?" For me a feeling, just that one tiny event of a synapse firing, can be the difference between a very fine day or a trip to the hospital.

On the day of my biggest reality check I was nineteen and having a very fine day indeed. I was earning a couple hundred dollars each shift as a night waitress, and had just landed a position working days as the assistant manager of a Vanity clothing store. I lived with my sister, Heather, and her husband, Marty. We were having a game night and sleepover with my two nephews, then eight and six years old, and my current boyfriend. Nothing felt better than finally being this normal.

Flash forward about five hours and I was in the emergency room, with vomit pouring out of my mouth and nose. I was anxious and angry and sick. Meanwhile a very rude doctor poked his fat face into my field of (blurry) vision and insisted on knowing what had happened.

To which I replied (with my trademark smartass grin), "I'm a little too busy to fuckin' talk right now."

Every person there wanted answers from me, and I just didn't have them. All I am certain of is that around midnight my entire world imploded. The façade I had so carefully built was demolished and even now, over a decade later, I am not entirely sure what happened. When I close my eyes I see handfuls of pills, but it is never me there in the cabinet mirror—it's someone else. Like watching a bad horror flick where the heroine runs up the stairs as you scream, "Stop! Don't go that way!" Unfortunately my inner voice screaming and pounding on that murky window didn't get through and I watched myself overdose on a bad movie. It wasn't me who mumbled things to my boyfriend as he ran to my sister's bedroom. It wasn't me being half carried down the nightmarishly long hallway of our apartment building. It wasn't me who rode in the car. It wasn't me until a rather large nurse roughly poured ipecac down my throat.

The fear of having my stomach pumped slapped me into reality and I began frantically shouting, "Please don't shove that tube up my nose!" In hindsight, that was definitely the wrong choice. I spent about an hour depositing the contents of my stomach into one of those little kidney-shaped dishes. Why on earth, with all the advances in medical science, haven't they realized that those things do not collect; they *splash*.

When I was stable enough to be moved, the large angry nurse dumped me into a wheelchair and carted me off to the intensive care room assigned to me. While I was being tucked into my rock hard adjustable bed I asked the nurse where my sister was. She had brought me in. I *needed* her.

As she unabashedly pulled off my shirt to hook me up to a heart monitor she gruffly stated, "Left. Not sure where. Your parents will be here in a couple hours."

Before this moment I had tried to keep a certain amount of self-deprecating humor about the whole situation to keep the panic at bay. Even as I dry-heaved I laughed a half hysterical giggle. I figured if I could treat it like a bad joke then it wouldn't hurt as much to know that I couldn't trust myself. But now my sister and even the mean nurse had abandoned me. Soon my parents would arrive and I knew the worst part would be looking into their eyes, because they wouldn't say a word.

That was when the tears started. That was when reason knocked on the door to my mind and demanded to be let back in. A feeling that can only be called shame, but which feels exponentially worse, overwhelmed me. I lay on my hard bed and sobbed, even louder and harder than I had cried when my father died. I was guilty, and sorry, but mostly I was angry because my very own mind had betrayed me. This had been a good day. A simple, honest good day and I just couldn't fathom what had suddenly gone wrong in my head. The fact that my body had done things that I didn't directly command it to do was tearing me apart. Who can you trust if you can't trust yourself?

I felt trapped in that shitty bed with stupid itchy electrodes stuck all over me, all the while suffering the nasty, judgmental looks from the staff members. As I stared at the blank television screen mounted on the wall across from me, my eyelids began to feel like someone had tucked lead weights into them. Then a strange thing happened. I saw, in the reflection of that TV, all the people I had ever known and loved. I don't know if it was the drugs still lingering in my system, or some strange spiritual warning, but I could see their faces giving me disapproving looks. Some scowled while others shook their heads or wiped away phantom tears. I saw ex-boyfriends, dead relatives, old friends—everyone. I was terrified and miserable laying in that cold hard bed surrounded by the disinfected hospital smell and the ghosts of my past. It was the most isolating moment of my entire life.

I assumed my heart would never ache like that again, but I was so wrong. When my parents crept into the room it was about 3:00 a.m. and they quietly sat down, trying not to wake me. I heard the rustle of their thick winter coats and the shuffle of their boots. I hadn't slept at all, but I closed my eyes and hid under the starchy blankets anyway. All I wanted was for my mother to cradle me like she had when I was small, to hear the whisper of, "It's alright, Sunshine." I wanted my stepfather to yell at me and tell me how stupid I was. But I knew they wouldn't. As I sat up in bed my mother looked at me with puffy eyes and whispered one word, "Why?"

It hurt. I felt the sting of that little word like the crack of a whip. I could tell by the look in her eyes she blamed herself, as if loving me wasn't quite enough. My stepfather couldn't even look at me; he sat stiffly in the corner, watching the snowflakes outside dance toward the ground. I squinted my eyes shut and wished I could become a particle of snow and be far removed from this room. Wishing didn't work; it just made the throbbing in my head worse. The three of us sat like that for most of the night.

Near dawn, my stepfather cleared his throat and reached into his coat pocket. He gently pulled out a slightly crumpled bouquet of fake white roses, the kind I guess you find at a gas station whilst speeding along in the middle of the night toward a disaster. The tag said, "For Someone Special," and inside he had simply written my name, like he wanted to remind me I was indeed important enough to inhabit the world. To date it was the biggest emotional gesture he had ever attempted with me and I was deeply touched. I tried my best to explain what had happened but I fully admit that the phrase, "I wasn't trying to kill myself. I just don't know what happened!" falls a bit short.

The doctors recommended a treatment center "for people like me" (I still resent them for using that type of language), and threatened to take away my rights as an adult. However, my mother fought tenaciously to have me released to her custody. I would go back to my childhood home, and back to my old counselor, so that they could all keep an eye on me. Nothing is more frustrating than wanting to be left alone when several people have appointed themselves your babysitter.

I went to my apartment to pack my things, tried to explain to Heather and Marty (once again falling short of the right words), and had to go quit my two jobs. I was torn out of the happy life I was building and carried back to the big house in the small town I had fought to get away from. Weeks after I had settled in, people were still giving me *the look,* my parents were still treating me like a child, and I was still blaming myself.

It took a long time to figure out what went wrong, but I have learned that occasionally things have to fall completely apart in order for you to rebuild an even stronger life for yourself. In the year spent back at home, I was able to repair and work through things with my parents and purge ghosts from my past. I worked, went to counseling, and then eventually went back to school. Had I never fallen apart I would never have met my best friend in college, forgiven my parents for mistakes of the past, or discovered amazing untapped strength within myself. I better understand the nature of my illness, and instead of fighting it, I treat it wisely and dance around it. I was broken, but became whole—and I still have the gas station roses on my bedside to remind me that, even on my darkest day, I am still "Someone Special".

*Carin Anderson is married to the love of her life, Jesse, and is the mom to her wonderful four year old son Leonidus. She was diagnosed with Bipolar Disorder at the age of 15. She spent the next ten years searching for the right medical team who has now helped her live her life on a balanced path with the right coping skills and medication. With the support of her big loud amazing family she has found peace in life and enjoys her many hobbies of being a musician, singer, songwriter, and a writer. She is most happy to just be herself.*

# THE FISH BOWL

## Katie Hiener

I open the door and look down the long driveway. A small, stone bridge stands at the end of the road ensuring only a single car can cross over the murky pond at a time. It's funny how that bridge signifies so much to me.

Five years ago I crossed the bridge to the safety of my home, and with the exception of an emergency trip to the hospital to remove my appendix, I had yet to cross back over. This disorder is called Agoraphobia, which literally means a "fear of the market place." Perhaps, at the time of definition, no one could realize there would be a zillion places to fear, not just a market.

Panic is a terrible thing and panic, in and of itself, can be feared. "Fear of the fear," is the name of that syndrome. And I had both.

My first attack was while driving. An overwhelming sense of doom swept through my psyche like a wave pummeling upon the shore. Powerful, intense, and—dear God—horrifying, I felt frightened, dizzy, nauseous, and had crushing chest pain. My initial thought was, *I'm dying.*

I managed to pull the car to the side of the road. I seemed destined to face mortality alone; it was in the pre-cell phone days. I shook, vomiting out the open car door as sweat poured down my entire body. I gasped for breath, held onto to the steering wheel, and prayed for the first time in my adult life.

The attack passed. I lived. I finished the drive home, somehow. Two shots of my dad's bourbon later I went to the blessed state called denial. I rationalized I had a stomach bug. Case closed.

But the devil was perched on one shoulder holding on tight. I had anxiety attacks everywhere: the post office, the grocery store, visiting a friend, eating at a restaurant. No place was safe. My excuses to flee the scene became clever, yet disproportionately ridiculous. I half believed myself as I lied about having the flu, a migraine, a backache, and allergies to everything. Learning to sense the onset of panic, I ran before it escalated.

I hid. I avoided the post office, stores, restaurants, and friends. Over time, I became a recluse, feeling safe and calm only in my home. My ignorant but well-meaning parents bought into the litany of physical ailments, and after many visits to a myriad of specialists we all seemed to accept that I had a mysterious illness. Home I stayed.

My folks went on with their lives and I pretended to live. Oh, I watched television, read avidly, and painted on canvas. My paintings were often ugly, always dark; I knew in the recesses of my mind that they reflected much more than my mood. The years passed. Some days I felt the weight of depression and other days I fantasized about taking my own life. I was truly living in hell.

I can't say what it was that shook my father into action, only that one day an extraordinarily tall man was in our living room. His quiet voice was close to a whisper and I found him enthralling. I remember his words, "Agoraphobia, it is an illness where panic leads to avoidance and that leads to a type of self-imprisonment. It is like you are a goldfish in a bowl."

I crossed the bridge with that man, a psychiatrist, who encouraged me to seek help.

After four months in a psychiatric hospital, I found that a combination of medication and therapy three times a week were in order. The program was geared toward people with phobias and through the sessions I learned I was not alone. We met in groups to share our hopes and our strengths. Slowly, my boundaries broadened.

I was anxious as my psyche healed. Crossing bridges both physically and metaphorically is no easy feat. I am mentally mending as I journey forward in life. The confines of my mind can no longer keep me inside of a fishbowl. I think often of a quote by Stephen Richards from *Releasing You from Fear* "When you have mastered fear then you have mastered all."

*Katie Hiener is a freelance writer with many passions. Animal Rights, Psychology and the Art of Story Telling find her with fingers flying over a keyboard. She is a featured writer for* Women Make Waves, *a private California Rehab, and the* Brookfield Patch. *Ms. Hiener also dreams of winning the lottery. If she is ever so lucky, you will find her running animal sanctuaries from her baby-blue Jeep, pen in hand, of course!*

# SHIT HAPPENS, RIGHT?

## Andrea Keeney

Just one year ago, in the final days of summer, I ventured out to the grocery store with my twelve-month-old daughter, Lizzie, and my two-year-old daughter, Melanie. The store was crowded and the only things keeping my daughters from a shopping cart seat breakout were a large box of crackers and two juice boxes. I weaved my way through the long aisles as fast as the large crowds would allow. As I rounded the corner of the bread aisle, my two-year-old daughter suddenly stopped chewing her mouthful of crackers.

"Mommy," she exclaimed. Several cracker crumbs flew out of her mouth and landed on the shopping cart. "I have to go pee-pee!"

"You do? Are you sure?" I asked only because my daughter was prone to potty false-alarms.

She nodded her head several times. "Yes, mommy. I really have to go!"

She wasn't kidding. I could tell by the serious look in her little blue eyes. Since she was just getting used to the feeling of having to go potty, there was a large chance that her bladder was extremely full and possibly ready to burst. I had to find a bathroom and quick, no matter how much I didn't want to.

Public restrooms were my own personal hell. They were oversized petri dishes of viruses and bacteria that were just waiting to hop aboard my germ-free body and infiltrate my immune system—or so my obsessive-compulsive disorder told me.

At one point, when my obsessive-compulsive disorder had just begun, I stayed a safe distance from all germ infested public restrooms. But that was before I had children—children who were potty training and pooping in diapers as we walked through the grocery store, the zoo, the museum, or whatever other public area they deemed the perfect locale to eliminate bodily waste.

Entering the small grocery store bathroom was like walking into a blanket of smells. The thick scent of an unventilated restroom, mixed with the faint scent of chemicals, smacked me in the face. Reflexively, I held my breath as I parked the cart in the largest stall and prayed I had the lung capacity to survive.

I helped Melanie to the toilet. Before her bottom reached the toilet seat she began to pee, spraying urine onto her underpants and down her legs. I pushed her further back onto the seat, stopping her from drenching the floor with urine.

"Mommy! I'm wet!" she squealed.

"I know," I snapped, helping her off the toilet.

I pulled the wet clothes from her tiny legs and redressed her with dry clothes. I was just moments from escaping the germ infested room when I caught the unpleasant smell of baby poop. I sighed, letting the air out of my lungs as I extracted a diaper, wipes, and a disposable changing pad from the bag. I pulled down the baby changing station, wiped it, and covered it with the protective pad. I wanted to wrap it with cellophane to keep my child from touching any part of the overused tray. With the fully sanitized station prepared, I placed Lizzie on the changing table. I set about removing her diaper and wiping her when suddenly, from behind me, I heard a rustling noise.

I looked back to see Melanie shuffling through the diaper bag. She had extracted a small bag of crackers and was set to start feasting. She stood very still, placing one cracker into her mouth after another. Then suddenly, for an unknown reason, she turned the bag upside down and shook it. Crackers fell to the floor, scattering in every direction. I knew what was going to happen next. I cringed and thought, *Holy cow, please no! Do not even think of it!* But it happened; my daughter dropped to the floor, grabbed a cracker, and shoved it in her tiny mouth.

"Melanie! No! Do not eat those off the floor. It is dirty!"

"No it's not mommy," she laughed.

"Yes, it is. Bathroom floors are dirty."

She smiled and laughed again, as if ingesting germs was comical.

*Not dirty*, I thought. I couldn't believe what she'd said. Didn't all people, even very small children, understand that floors—especially bathroom floors—were covered in germs? Influenza, Herpes, Ebola, Salmonella, basically every deadly disease that could be thought of. They were all in here incubating and just waiting for a little child's hand to pick up a germ ridden cracker and gobble it up it; or at least I thought they were.

"Just leave the crackers," I sighed. "I will pick them up when I am done with your sister."

I turned back to Lizzie. She grinned mischievously as she tossed one chubby leg over her body and tried to roll free from my grasp. I caught her, but she began to squirm even more. She kicked her diaper, sending the fully loaded package across the changing table and onto my shirt. My daughter kicked again, this time smashing the dirty diaper against me. I could feel the warm poop squish onto my shirt. I reached down and pulled the diaper off of me. A large brown circle remained, the mark of motherhood emblazoned on me. To my horror, my daughter kicked again, shoving her toe into the diaper. She yanked her foot back. Poop flew through the air. It seemed to linger above her for a long moment before it came back down. It splattered on her white shirt, just above her belly.

I froze. I may have been medicated for obsessive-compulsive disorder, but not even my high dose of Prozac could contain my reaction to flying bowel movements. I wanted to vomit. Actually, I wanted to run screaming from the bathroom and saturate my children with soap and warm water. Instead, I took a deep breath and finished wiping my daughter's bottom. I removed her poop-stained shirt and re-dressed her in the spare outfit I'd brought. I rolled the diaper up and placed it in an extra plastic bag before strapping Lizzie back into the shopping cart seat.

When I turned to gather my other daughter she was not where I expected her to be. Instead of standing in the center of the stall she was on her hands and knees, attempting to escape under the locked door. My stomach clenched in horror, my mind raced, and my mouth dropped open.

"Melanie. I just told you that the floor is dirty!"

"But I'm not eating."

Touché, I thought. "Please stand up."

Melanie complied, but sighed loudly to announce her annoyance. We stopped at the sink in hopes of removing the poop from my shirt and the dozens of germs that were surely lingering on Melanie's hands. As we were elbow deep in scrubbing, a middle-aged woman walked into the restroom and stopped at the sink beside me. She adjusted her hair, then made eye contact with me in the mirror. She looked down at my shirt and wrinkled her nose.

"Sorry for the smell," I said quietly. "We had a little diaper mishap."

The woman grinned and looked at my daughters. Then she leaned in close to me, lowered her voice to a whisper, and summed up the entirety of my restroom catastrophe in one phrase.

"Hey, shit happens, right?"

*Andrea Keeney is a chef, driver, booger-wiper, master of dance parties, laundry expert, and CEO of family affairs. In short, she is a mother and wife. When she isn't navigating the rough terrain of parenting, she is writing. Andrea is the author of the hilarious book,* Moms: As Elite as the CIA...Well Almost, *as well as the creator of the blog* Parenting with Parents.

# THE ATTACK

## Veronica Leigh

It often surprises me, usually when I am completely unaware and having fun. I could be spending an hour at the library looking for books, or out to eat with my family, or even at church. Wherever I am, I am in my own little world when it strikes. This particular time I am at Walmart shopping for clothes. I riffle through the rack of blouses, obliviously enjoying myself. I don't see it coming, don't feel it creeping up on me.

I am unaware of its presence until it slips out from the shadows and is hovering near my shoulder, hissing taunts in my ear. I duck my head, in hopes of eluding it. My eyes scan the area; I must distract myself. If I let it overcome me, I will once again be the victim. I frantically tear through the clothing, agitated that my plan doesn't seem to be working, and move on to the next part of the store: the movies. I must get my mind on something else, and fast! It stalks me, a darkness intent on wholly engulfing me. The darkness held me captive for almost a decade. I know I must fight it.

As I pass by a shelf, my hand automatically shoots out to touch it. I touch a pole next and then an abandoned shopping cart. I chuckle to myself.

"You're like Adrian Monk," my sister has told me time and time again. "You touch things as you walk past them."

Of all my quirks, touching things had to be one of my funniest. At least I could laugh about it. It does distract me from my current struggle.

I begin to pray, begging God to help me hold it together.

I slip my hand into my pocket and clutch my lucky crucifix, or as I call it, my "Pocket Jesus." Deep down I know the crucifix does not shield me from it. But it provides me comfort. That's something I need.

Though I am strengthened by my crucifix, I am still shaky. I need to check out. Heading into the main aisle at the front of the store, the wide, white open space, I begin to feel my body temperature rise. This is how it always starts; it used to end with me in tears, fleeing to my comfort zone.

I cough. Sometimes the terror makes my throat feel swollen even though it's not. I break out into a sweat. Okay, it is now sinking its sharp claws into me, determined to tear into me and leave its mark. My heart is beating faster and faster. I am beginning to feel dizzy as the room whirls around me.

I grasp the necklace dangling from my neck and fiddle with it. Yes, another one of my quirks. I always wear necklaces and I am always messing with them. Don't get me started on how many I have broken and blamed their flimsy chains because I was flustered.

I am almost there! If I can manage a little longer, I will make it.

It makes one last attempt to break me: a wave of nausea hits me full force. Usually this is a last measure and it doesn't often use it, but this time it is close to succeeding.

I reach the counter, mumble a few words of small talk, and pay for my items. It feels like eternity but somehow I make it without fainting or dropping into the fetal position on the cold linoleum. I pass through the sliding doors and to my car with my head held high; triumph and pride fills me. This time I survived the attack and am able to go throughout the day as if nothing happened.

It slinks away in defeat. But I know it is plotting its next attack. Until then, I am victorious over my anxiety attacks. I vow to not let them make me a victim any longer. I cannot go back; I will never go back. I place my hand in my pocket and caress the crucifix. My breathing returns to normal and I reach out to touch the light pole

*Veronica lives with her mother, sister, aunt, and six furbabies in Indiana. She continues to have anxiety attacks but has found a way to live despite them. She dreams of becoming a published novelist and has been published in three other anthologies. You can find out more about her on her blog Veronica Leigh.*

# THROW ME A ROPE

## Angila Peters

Six years ago the world around me shifted when my second child arrived, a son. Instead of the joyous afterglow of a newborn in my arms I slipped, quietly and secretly, from sanity to a total detachment from logic.

He wasn't a difficult child, but attending to a new baby with a shadow looming was difficult. A heavy darkness was seeping into my mothering heart and I wouldn't have recognized it if it shook my hand and said its name. However, the darkness was shaking me deeply and altering my thinking, reality, and mind.

My husband owned his own business, and we lived in a small, remote village with no family nearby. In fact our whole family lived on the other side of the country, which left us with little support or extra hands. We were in debt and couldn't take too much time off, but all would be well, I thought. We could do this—until I couldn't do this.

When you have a newborn there isn't time to sit and ponder about being overwhelmed. Everyone on Earth (it seems) has raised children and made it, so at first I told myself I would be fine. People around me kept telling me how lucky, blessed, and strong I was with that look of awe in their eyes. My daughter was an amazing big sister; the baby was healthy and handsome. Who could complain about that? But I felt alone, so very alone.

It turns out I was a perfect candidate for postpartum depression (PPD), because doctors had already diagnosed me with general anxiety disorder. Denial is how I dealt with the diagnoses. I brushed off the doctors as pill pushers and dug my feet deep into the ground. Strong, sane people don't need medication. I focused my energies on reading self-help books, exercising, and ignoring. None of it worked.

I focused on living out the preconceived story I had imagined. I was going to be a great, happy, wonderful mother. My first-born was an easy child, a textbook dream, and after she was born I was fine and happy, like a good mama—or so I believed. Preparing for my son's birth wasn't in my plans since I had been there, done that. Except each birth is different, and I hadn't planned on that either.

The area in which we lived did not offer birthing services at all, so like any local pregnant family we had to leave town, pay for accommodations, and secure a delivery team. We rented a vacation home in another city and finished our last prenatal visits there until the baby came.

Having to travel three hours to give birth uprooted our little family. It cost a lot of money and caused stress I didn't need. Whereas my first child was born in a hospital with an epidural and a team of helpers, the second was born in less than an hour, in a rental home, with a panicked midwife and no drugs. My labor was fast and furious with no break. I remember feeling like a caged cat that was about to die.

I'd been expecting and secretly hoping for another girl, but out came my son—ten-and-a-half pounds of baby boy. My mind was already trying to process: *How do I take care of a boy?* I looked at my husband and a tinge of guilt flushed my face for actually being upset it was a boy. I was caught off guard because I love my boys (I've had a third child, a son, since this episode with PPD), but at the moment I was scared.

Once we made it back to our village with a healthy son, I fully expected motherhood bliss to envelop me. Instead I was angry, exhausted, and sick. While everyone was celebrating, I was trying not to drown. I wanted both help and independence. I longed to prove I was a good mother but I was failing.

Secrets are hard to keep, and I was having a difficult time hiding my self-destruction. The only person I had to confide in was my husband. Begging him to take over, knowing something wasn't right, became our daily conversation. I suffered through every agonizing second he was away from me. He needed to run our business, our family's source of income; I needed to crawl inside a hole and die. My husband was forced to accept the role of mother to us all. He worked, came home, cooked, cleaned and kept the shit together. He pressed repeat and so did I, with no end in sight.

The only release came when I let my anger out. The problem was that I directed my frustrations at my kids and myself. I would yell at the baby to please sleep. He would cry, and I would be awash in shame. Our beautiful daughter would innocently want attention and I would scream for her to have a nap. I just needed five minutes of quiet—just five—but there was no peace.

I was beyond sleep deprived and with a feeling of total defeat, I snapped. At some point, on some day, I slammed my bedroom door and started punching myself in the head. What kind of a mother yells at her perfectly innocent kids? What sane person hits her own head with her fists? Coming undone felt inevitable, but self-harm was a new low for me. Punching my head felt like the punishment I deserved for being such an asshole to my babies. I called myself horrible names and threatened to turn myself in to the police. But the threat of being known to the outside world for my faults kept me hidden.

One night my illness told me to get on a bus. Just leave. I was the worst mother in the world, and the only obvious solution was to give my family the gift of my absence. I convinced myself that they would be better without me. Not once did it occur to me they would miss me. In fact, I felt I owed it to them to stop the craziness I was bringing into the house. We were all miserable. They were walking on eggshells and all I could do was exist in a pile of defeat.

Standing in front of the bathroom mirror, I looked at the woman reflected back at me and said, "You fucking, ungrateful bitch. Don't you dare yell at those kids ever again! Get out! Go now. It's the least you can do. Fucking idiot." I smiled back at her. Finally someone was telling the truth. I punched my head harder than before, to make sure I got the message crystal clear, and started packing my overnight bag. I was frighteningly calm.

I had started gathering my necessities for living alone when I saw my nipple cream. I paused. Will I need it? My next thought was, *I'm his source of food.* Fuck.

I crawled into a corner of the bathroom where I rocked myself back and forth. *This is crazy. This is how going insane feels.* I moaned, like a contraction was hitting my body at full force. I was weeping and moaning. *I want on that bus, but I can't even do that. Yelling is one thing, but starving my baby? No. I need fucking help.*

I don't know where I found the number, or how long I talked. I just know the woman on the end of the line saved me. She saved my soul. She told me to get a washcloth, soak it in water and spend the next ten minutes wringing it out with my hands. She waited on the other end. It felt amazing. Anger ripped and wrenched the cloth. She called me normal, and said she would give me tools. I agreed to not leave the house or get on a bus.

I've never written about my time in the dark because I still feel the pain. I am not completely recovered, even seven years later. My son's first year is a total blank. So much time was consumed in my distorted mind with self-loathing, that I missed the good.

Sometimes I still feel haunting guilt and shame, especially when my son asks what his life was like then. Part of me wants to hide the truth so he never knows I yelled or wished him motherless. It had nothing to do with him. Depression, anxiety, and PPD robbed us both that year. And honestly, my mental illnesses still take front stage sometimes. It never goes away. It's just more controlled, for which I am forever grateful.

Thankfully, while my husband was busy keeping us all together he was videotaping precious moments, moments otherwise lost to me. Those clips are a gift. Memories of my first and third children hold strong because I was present. My middle one not so much.

Forgiveness happens when I am kind to myself. I use writing, humor, and sharing to heal as well. Whenever someone owns their story of suffering I can sit and listen, like the woman on the phone. I was very lucky that day. I know that, and I pay it forward whenever the opportunity arises.

*Angila is a freelance writer based in Southern Ontario, Canada. She has written for many platforms, and covered different genres. She is a featured writer for* Blunt Moms, *and can be found on* Huffington Post *as well. Angila shares humorous stories about mental health issues, current events, and parenting on her blog* Detached From Logic.

# UDDERLY HILARIOUS

## Tricia Stream

B reastfeeding was an absolute no-go when it came to tiny, 2-pound persons who weren't even capable of remembering to breathe on their own. But when the neonatal intensive care unit (NICU) staff told me breast milk was liquid gold for preemies, I embarked upon a very intimate relationship with my pump—like a human participant in one of Mike Rowe's *Dirty Jobs* episodes on dairy farming with Holstein cows.

I've fought depression and anxiety for over a decade. I'll find myself struggling with "episodes" when they sneak up on me if I'm not paying attention. I don't think you'd really notice by looking at me; I can still appear to be fully functional to those merely observing my superficial exterior. Yet when my twin boys made their appearance into the world thirteen weeks too soon—several days shy of the start of the third trimester—I couldn't be bothered with my own mental health. I reasoned I wasn't susceptible to postpartum depression because I was already depressed. Besides, I didn't have time for baby blues; I focused solely on my sons' survival, namely by strapping an industrial grade suction apparatus to two of the most sensitive areas of my body and trying to literally squeeze the life out of them.

The biggest challenge to face was the loss of control. No matter how involved in the babies' care, no matter how much time I spent the NICU or how much juju I thought I had to spare, I had trouble accepting the full loss of control—over my sons' health or my own mind. Zero, zip, zilch. I went through the motions every day. But there were fleeting moments when I'd stare through the kitchen window, out into the emptiness of a sunlit suburban street, while scrubbing my breast milk accouterments and wonder if it was worth it. Did I even want to be a mother anymore?

Finally a month later, when my sons were comfortably cocooned as burrito babies of the in-between (the period of time after preemies are born, but before homecoming) at the ripe old age of negative two months, I forced aside my guilt of being away from their hospital isolettes for more than the requisite thirty minutes every three hours spent in the "Mothers Room" and accepted a lunch date. Three of my girlfriends managed to convince me that they were really interested in seeing me and dammit, we were going out.

About halfway through my third glass of ice water (a lot of hydration goes into the dairy farming process), the restaurant suddenly became colder than the Arctic Circle during a particularly frigid cold spell. I pushed the water away and clutched at the chips left from our salsa and queso appetizer in hopes of salvaging some of their radiating, microwaved heat. I tore into a molten lava cake, searing my tongue with the scalding chocolate.

Ultimately I fled the restaurant to bask in the 85-degree California day, but it still wasn't warm enough. My car had been sitting out in July's summer sun all morning, so the interior temperature was probably about 115 degrees; it was almost warm enough, but only with the heater on. Once home, because of the shady tree overhanging our house, I immediately pulled on every sweatpant- and sweatshirt-like piece of clothing I could find and climbed under the covers of my bed. I had a fever of 103.

Teeth chattering, I called the NICU to let them know I wouldn't be in for the boys' evening bath. Sick people are strictly forbidden in that particular hospital unit—for obvious reasons. Nurses assured me the boys were still doing great and that I should get some rest and take care of myself (i.e. don't come infect any fragile babies). Then a nurse offhandedly asked how the pumping was going.

"Is there pain or a burning sensation while you pump?"

Well, pumping sucked—but it had pretty much been like that from the very beginning. *You* try attaching two large suction cups to rather delicate areas of your body and turning on a vacuum. Of course there was pain and burning.

"Swollen breasts?"

That was a definite affirmative. Silly me, I'd figured that was a result of the whole being filled with milk thing. It was visually apparent by the nursing bra I wore, which looked like two prairie bonnets from the days of the Oregon Trail.

"The bad news is," the nurse continued with her diagnosis, "I think you have mastitis. It usually occurs within the first twelve to fourteen days of breastfeeding. Try taking a very hot shower and massaging yourself."

That sounded like a lot of work. I just wanted to curl up into a little ball and die. And also, no one was getting near my boobs, myself included. But get near them I would. Despite my feverish hallucinations, I continued to wake up every three hours for intimate relations with my pump before collapsing again. My husband was also less than thrilled that the prescribed treatment involved breast massages in a hot shower and he wasn't invited. I was heartbroken at having to throw good food, literally, down the drain.

The next day I decreed myself well enough to head back to the hospital. At first I thought it was simply relief that both boys were relatively healthy, but I quickly realized my flush of relief was the return of my fever. The thought of holding either boy seemed utterly exhausting. The lavender walls, chosen for their calming color, were closing in around me. The isolettes oscillated in my mind while the reams of wires swayed back and forth in a hypnotic fashion. I had to find a doctor.

In a haze, I made my way to the clinic. At 4:45 p.m., and without an appointment, I stumbled up to the registration desk. "My boobs are infected, I think. I don't feel good. Can I see a doctor? I probably need drugs," I announced to the world at large.

The receptionist told me to "sit tight" and disappeared into the back to "see what she could do." This was meant to reassure me that she was searching for medical help, though she was likely calling security. Especially after she asked me for my insurance identification card. Which I did not have. Because it was in my purse, containing my proof of person, which remained back in the hallowed walls of the NICU.

The medical assistant, who came out to see what was going on, highly encouraged me to go away and come back tomorrow during office hours (or when someone other than her would have to deal with me). I'm not sure whether it was my sudden outburst of sobs or collapsing to the ground clutching my swollen breasts, but I was pretty sure the world was about to end. Ultimately, the medical assistant took pity on me (or she realized I was fully prepared to cause a scene to be remembered).

I was escorted into the back room. An annoyed looking nurse pointed at a chair in her office and threatened me with the adult version of the pulse oximeter. For the saner sort, this is nothing more than a clip fitted over one's index finger, where it emits a glowing red light. For me, it was the sole representation of the preemie struggle. I had a PTSD response to the high-pitched beeps that replicated the tones of monitoring alarms in the NICU—what if my children's oxygen stats plummeted while I blithely had my own measured?

She jabbed a thermometer under my tongue.

"You have a fever."

"I know."

"103."

"I don't feel good."

I removed my shirt. There was no hesitation here. I would likely have removed the shirt even if I'd still been in the lobby. Or the parking lot. Everybody and anybody gets a show if they can *just fix it*.

My babies were sick and my boobs hurt.

"Wow. Your breasts are very swollen," said the nurse stuck dealing with me. "You need to be breastfeeding more. Every hour."

I burst into tears. The fever was fueling my anxiety. The hamster in my brain was amped up like an addict high on a cocktail of speed and Red Bull. My muscles took matters into their own hands, tensing up to the point of pain. I was shaking now, trembling in fear from the terrible, awful "what if."

Anxiety is totally normal. It's a human defense mechanism to get a little fidgety and need to take a deep breath when dealing with a stressful situation. Just chill out. Easier said than done. Especially when your mind has embarked upon an Oscar caliber creative endeavor to convince you that everything can (and will) go wrong. Anxiety is more than just a twinge of unease; it is a full-fledged fight-or-flight response. Unfortunately you're the only one in your way—it's not easy to escape yourself and it's never healthy to harm yourself (or the medical professional tasked with talking you down).

I explained that I couldn't breastfeed. My sons weren't old enough to suck, swallow, and breathe. The nurse eyed me with intense skepticism, clearly thinking I did not understand how babies worked. Amid sobs and between gasps for breath, which really made me sound like a depressed barking seal, I managed to somehow convey the concept that I had preemies presently focused more on getting their tiny bodies to, you know, make blood, than they were on my boobs.

In my expert (read: hysterical) opinion, this was far more impor- tant than even considering when the timing would be right to shove a boob in their mouth. Especially given said boob was currently larger than their little heads.

It took a bit more prompting, as Nurse Irritable attempted to pro- cess how someone not breastfeeding had managed to get mastitis. It all came down to the intimate bonding relationship motherhood had given me with my Medela Breast Pump and its soothing, sucking, wooshing. So pumping every hour was the simple solution?

I did the math in my feverish mind. Three minutes to gather equipment, five minutes to prep the pump and various accou- terments, a minute to attach pump suction-y things to my body, pump for fifteen minutes, bag and label the liquid gold, and five minutes dutifully scouring all the pump parts for next time. A 30-minute process, which I'd have to start all over again thirty minutes later.

This would give me a half hour out of each hour to live my life. I may as well just have the damn thing attached to my udders 24/7. I was fully dedicated to procuring this life-saving liquid that all the nurses kept congratulating me on. But I was exhausted, mentally and physically.

I could hear my pulse loudly drumming in my ears; I had a strange sensation of blood coursing through my veins. My mind went blank as I attempted to breathe in pathetically shallow, conscious puffs. Breathe in. Breathe out. Breathe in. Breathe out. Remember to keep doing this. Suddenly I was keenly aware of what my tiny ones were facing.

The pressure and stress of those NICU months, combined with my feverish realization that my pumping problems were only going to get worse, conspired to trigger a massive anxiety attack. But some- how, with my little babies depending on me, I was able to focus on what I needed to do.

I looked up, my swollen boobs still flashed to the world, and mooed at the nurse in frustration.

My point was made.

*Corporate writer by day, mommy blogger by night, Tricia is a Silicon Valley tech geek raising twin toddlers – Search and Destroy. Instead of having one baby after 9 months, she had two after 6; she's efficient like that. She has dealt with depression and anxiety for over a decade and shares her stories far and wide on her blog* Stream of the Conscious, *because the only way to survive is to find the humor of the situation.*

# THE MOMENT THE PANIC BEGAN

## Alyson Herzig

I used to be someone, I used to be able to do something, and then it changed. It wasn't a gradual shift; I know the exact moment it changed, right down to the second. I can transport myself, without even trying, to the minute when it slipped through my fingers.

I was twenty-six years old and a supervisor of twenty male truck drivers. I was young and naive, but also stubborn and proud. I learned the Department of Transportation regulations. I memorized and understood the union contract. I spent time studying the specifications of their trucks, the contracts for the equipment, the driver routes, the pricing, all of it—no stone left unturned. I plunged head-on into it because I never wanted to be in a situation where my lack of knowledge impacted others' opinions of my capabilities.

One day an employee, whose dislike for me was visible and who made every possible attempt to ensure I knew it, refused to run a route he was assigned. It was not his normal route; it was a longer one, and he didn't want to drive it. He stood against the white, painted concrete wall and looked down at me from his towering height, gruffness oozing from his pores. He hid behind his union seniority. He did not realize I knew the rules of the contract and he could not refuse. I insisted he run the truck route and he begrudgingly complied, but afterward he filed a grievance with the union against me.

Whenever a grievance is filed it starts a paper trail and ultimately a meeting results between the plant human resources (HR) manager, the employee's manager, the employee, and the union representative. Both sides air their version of the complaint. I was prepared for the meeting like a Girl Scout, ready to discuss his behavior. It was me in a room of men, in a male-dominated company, in the male-run plant; I was the only woman.

I remember the room perfectly: the HR manager behind his large, old-school brown desk that gleamed with shellac and me against the wall in a 1980-style wooden chair that was slightly angled toward the door. Just to my left, no more than three feet away, was the union president. He was dressed in his grey work t-shirt, scuffed steel-toed boots, and stained blue jeans. His wiry salt and pepper hair framed his hard, worn face. Next to him was the employee who'd filed the grievance. He was dressed in nice, clean blue jeans and a pressed, short-sleeved, powder blue collared shirt buttoned up to the top button. His chair was blocking the door and was almost directly across from mine, giving us each a clear view of the other. Normally I would never remember the detail of someone's clothing, but this was a moment that would forever be imparted into my brain. I remember every single second of that meeting in intricate detail.

I presented my case and my side of the issue. I highlighted the contractual agreement the driver had with the company. I would be lying if I said the employee and the union president didn't intimidate me; they did, yet I stuck to my convictions and relied on my wits.

But then it happened—the moment that changed me. The instant when I went from being calm and collected in group settings to experiencing near crippling panic attacks that have held me captive for the last twelve years.

The union president jumped up from his seat and lunged toward me, his brow furrowed over his dark, age-worn eyes, spit spewing from his mouth as he yelled at me. His arm was outstretched in anger while he shouted his hatred. I held my spot in the chair, just staring at him, shocked at what was unfolding. The HR manager leapt from behind his desk, the employee sprang from his chair, all while I sat motionless. Speechless. The HR manager had grabbed the union president just before he attacked me and pulled him outside into the hallway to cool off. I continued to sit, just watching it unfold. It was then that I felt the first assault of panic. I struggled to maintain my composure, but my breath was spastic and a stabbing pain wrapped itself around my chest like a hawk's talon around its prey.

This was the exact moment I broke.

I do not know why my mind snapped. Maybe it was a lifetime of compartmentalizing every single thing and space just ran out.

Over the past twenty years I'd compartmentalized a lot of life changes. This work meeting may have tipped the scales, spilling all of my calm and composed control into chaos, but it did so with the weight of a lot of stressors.

Maybe it was the stress of relocating to a new state; my husband and I had moved a thousand miles from Dallas, TX where we had previously worked to Indiana for his job. In that time we'd also gotten married in my home state of New Jersey, and starting a life on new ground can be unsettling. Or was it my strained relationship with my parents that caused me to tip? Maybe building a new house was just too much for me to juggle. My life had gone from predictable monotony to complete upheaval in little under a year.

There are so many maybes; I will never know the answer. Most likely it is all of the above. It was a life of holding my breath in times of stress that had strangled my inner self. My psyche would not take one more thing hurled at it. My mind clamped down on that sunny, warm August day in 2001, and has not released itself since.

Sometimes my panic goes dormant, waiting to attack. I have stepped to the front of a room for a business presentation and been unable to breathe, going through my presentation slides in rapid succession in an attempt to end the pain as quickly as possible. When I had my first child I did not return to work. I was a relieved to never walk into the building again. Never having to stand in front of my peers unable to think or talk. I had hoped it was the end of the panic, but it wasn't.

Even outside the workplace, long since having left my job to be at home with my kids, I've been rendered paralyzed at the most inopportune moments. Important events I've attended with my husband where I'm forced to interact with people I'm unfamiliar with have left me struggling to find my composure. Often I've needed to take medication to make it through without a panic attack. Other times something as little as standing up and asking a question at an informational event at my children's school has left me unable to breathe. My heart races and I'm left shaking afterward. It is a horrible feeling that I wish on no one.

Of course, there is never a good time for a fear so deep that I am unable to breathe except in shallow breaths that terrorize me. But there are times when I can avoid it, triggers I can watch for. I have learned that crowded places are a major trigger for my anxiety. Speaking, reading, or leading discussions in front of others is a guaranteed stressor that sends my heart racing, my hands shaking, my throat closing. No amount of mental games will stop an attack once it starts. My only hope is heading it off before it begins. Medicine has helped to keep the attacks at bay; however, they have not been completely slayed.

Panic attacks are like a dragon, waiting in the shadows to come out and rip my soul apart, to breathe fire on my sanity, leaving my mind scorched and barren. I am left afraid and feeling inadequate. Each one seems so ridiculous after it happens, but at the time I am spiraling into an abyss I feel I may never escape.

The most recent attack happened at a major writing conference I attended. I foolishly stepped out of my comfort zone and signed up for a program that would have required me to be on stage pitching an idea to a group of literary agents. This was the whole reason I was at this conference. I desperately wanted to be selected to present my idea.

I spent weeks preparing for this moment, revising and rewriting my speech until it sung. I would not allow my panic to stop me from living; I could not allow it to win. So I sat in the audience and felt it creeping closer. I became more and more anxious as participants were selected. I watched the other attendees present their ideas and marveled at the ease with which they spoke. Some smiled, laughed, or acted out their ideas while I sat nailed to my chair, allowing the worry to come and grab a hold of my heart, squeezing it tight, tighter. The pains were deep, slicing into my body with each breath. Eventually my lungs could not expand. I was enveloped in a black sheath coiling around me.

I prayed I would be selected so I could prove to myself I could beat out the demon. I wanted to prove that I would win. But fate had a go at me and I was not selected. I was crestfallen. I allowed any remaining opportunity to slip through my hands and ran from that room as soon as it was over. I spent no time networking. I left as quickly as I could. I raced to the stairwell. I needed air, fresh air. I stood outside in the late afternoon light and watched the other attendees chat and revel in the experience. I stood in line for the bus to the hotel and realized I had to leave. I had to go home. Right then. There was no other option.

I left the conference and drove four hours home. The first two hours were a blur. I was distracted by my feelings of frustration and anger that I had once again allowed the beast to rise up inside me.

I allowed the panic to dictate my actions and override my sensibilities. I didn't say goodbye to anyone. I just left. I was fleeing from the moment, the place that triggered the attack. My only thought was *go home, I must go home.* The need was so strong; the only antidote to my pain was my home.

And then the beast went dormant again. So I wait. I wait for the next attack. Will I be stronger? Will I defeat the dragon that haunts me? After all I was someone, I used to be able to do things. But then it changed.

*Originally from NJ, Alyson now lives in the Midwest but has kept her sarcastic cynical Jersey attitude. You can find her blogging about the many disasters and observations of her life at her popular humor site* The Shitastrophy. *Alyson has had essays published in the anthology,* My Other Ex: Women's True Stories of Losing and Leaving Friends *as well as the anthology* Not Your Mother's Book: On Working for a Living, *and the follow up sequel* I Still Just Want to Pee Alone. *She has published pieces at* Huffington Post, Scary Mommy, What The Flicka, Mamapedia, *and other online venues.*

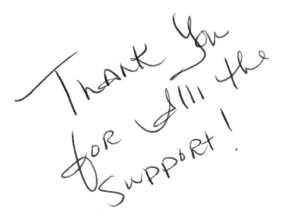

# HAPPINESS IS NOT A CHOICE
## Linda Roy

This morning I woke up with that familiar feeling. No, it wasn't a relaxed, well rested, greet-the-day-with-a smile-on-my-face feeling, it was more of a horrible, anxious, clenching-fist-in-the-pit-of-the-stomach feeling.

Some days it doesn't matter how good my life is or how relatively calm things are. Upon entering consciousness, pure dread and anxiety take over as soon as I open my eyes.

When this happens, it is a signal that the entire day, even before my feet touch the floor, will be a wash. I will be unmotivated, unable to think straight, irritable, impatient, unfocused, sad, angry, anxious—all of it. But why? When there is no particular weight pressing on me, no deadlines, no places to shuttle the kids to or unpaid bills to agonize over, why would I feel this way? The feeling seems to come out of nowhere to invade my mind and body like an emotional virus.

This virus is one that doesn't warrant a sick day in bed. It's not one that earns a pass from day-to-day responsibilities. Instead it's considered a weakness, a pity party, a form of self-absorption.

Doesn't anybody understand I can't help it?

No, they don't.

"Snap out of it! Happiness is a choice."

People living with depression hear that a lot. Oh, and of course it's always from people who don't get it.

"If you just wake up in the morning, put a smile on your face and make a conscious choice to be happy, you will be. And then others around you will be happy, and so on…"

And la-dee-da. Rainbows and unicorns will spew forth, perhaps ushering in the advent of world peace!

It's so simple. So why can't I do that? Oh yeah, depression.

I live with something called dysthymia. It is a low-grade form of chronic depression. It's mild, yet not mild enough to ignore. It forever hovers like the cloud over the little water droplet in the Zoloft commercials. It's so low grade, in fact, that the majority of people who suffer from it, experience it from childhood into adulthood entirely undetected and undiagnosed. Those are the moody kids.

I was the moody kid. My family didn't understand it, I'm sure many of my friends wondered why I was such a pain in the ass, and I preferred to glamorize it away as the product of my tortured, artistic existence. This was Emo before it was even a marketable entity. Oh, shit. I'm going to ignore that thought, lest I begin to wax apoplectic over lost opportunity and revenue.

The point is, I didn't know what was happening. I just knew I was sad a lot. And angry. And anxious. And I wore a lot of black.

Was it because my father died when I was eight? I'm sure that probably contributed to things. I remember my third grade teacher pulled me out of class one day and explained I would be going to a special group a couple of times a week. In this special group, we would just talk. About anything. We could talk about our lives at home, how we felt about school—whatever. At that young age, I wondered what could have possibly earned me the coveted "Get Out of Jail Free" card. But who cared? I got out of math class.

That first day walking into the school psychologist, Miss Veres's office, I saw a few of my classmates sitting at a table. They were people I considered to be artistic; one was into music and the other wanted to be a comedian. I wanted to be an actress and musician. I was always cracking jokes. Was this a deprogramming group for wayward artistic types?

Miss Veres looked like Merv Griffin in a wig and pumps. She was about forty-something with chin length salt and pepper hair that abruptly turned up at the jawline, rouge smeared onto her swarthy cheeks, and thick, muscular legs. During many of our sessions, she'd hike a heel up onto an open desk drawer, pull out a jack knife and sharpen a pencil by hand like Davy Crockett in a Chanel suit.

She never came right out and said, "Hey, you guys are all here because we've noticed you have emotional problems: you still suck your thumb, you lost your father, and you ... why are you here again?" Instead, we just talked. We cracked jokes, did impressions, and measured life's injustices, one sharpened pencil at a time. I never realized I was attending my first group therapy sessions.

Later on, I always assumed I had been there because my father died.

Looking back now, I remember my nursery school teacher advising my mother to seek counseling for me because I once stubbornly staged a sit-in under the craft table, refusing to color a picture of a bunch of grapes green (I wanted to color them purple) when the teacher insisted they should be green. Come to think of it, I tended to camp out under that table a lot. Did she see something in me even then? Some sort of connection to my depression that was overshadowed by the absurdity of the situation?

I waded through adolescence with the usual mother–daughter battles, a stepfather with whom I didn't get along, siblings to whom I couldn't relate, and increasing feelings of not belonging, never quite fitting in, and isolation. I attributed it to teenage angst and malcontent. I never put two and two together until I met my husband, who pointed out I was one angry, confrontational son-of-a-gun.

Despite a couple of failed attempts at a diagnosis from therapists who would only shrug, shake their heads, and announce, "It could be worse," I still knew something was not quite right. In their informed professional opinions, what I seemed to be experiencing was just the ups and downs of everyday life. Sure, I had endured some rough spots, but it just didn't seem normal to be so unhappy, so sad, so angry, so numb, so much of the time. At times the rage would build up inside me like Mount Vesuvius and the feeling wouldn't go away until I erupted all over anyone close enough to drown in my emotional lava.

At last I found a therapist who recognized my dysthymia almost immediately. She would always say that the first time I came into her office, I was so full of anger. I still have some of that anger. I think I always will. But now I know how to deal with it.

And medication? We are still guinea pigs, all of us who live with any form of mental illness. Does this pill work? Great! Try that for a year or two. Not doing it for you anymore? Try this one! No? Try this one *and* that one. I used to go to a ninety-five-year-old psychiatrist who would just ask me, "What are you taking and how much? What dosage do you want?" Then he'd look it all up in this little black book he kept in his desk drawer that's probably been there since 1952. I tried asking for Oxycontin once just to see if he was paying attention. That's the one time he was.

"You know that this can be habit forming, don't you?"

"Yes."

"Well, we don't want that, do we?"

"No?"

Actually, all I've ever really wanted was to be in the habit of being happy, of feeling normal, whatever that is.

Comedian Steve Martin used to say there were no sad banjo songs. Now, I'm a musician, and I'm a humorist, and I figured there must be something to that theory. So I went out and got myself a banjo. I figured that between the medication and the banjo, there was gonna be a whole lotta happy going on. I realized two things. The first is that if happiness were a choice, we'd all either learn to play banjo or we'd be loitering next to the log flume ride at Six Flags. And the second is that I'm probably the first person to ever write a dirge for the banjo.

On the plus side of depression, at least now that I know what I'm dealing with and how to manage it, I have fewer anxiety-riddled mornings, fewer volcanic eruptions, and a whole lot more motivation.

If happiness were a choice, if it really was as simple as making lemonade out of lemons, then my life would be all Lynchburg lemonades and banjo music on the front porch. But it's not a choice. Some of us have a chemical imbalance in our brains that causes us to live with various forms of mental illness. And to us, that's normal. And we get through it from one day to the next, with therapy, with meds, and with the support of those who mean the most to us. And also, with the occasional glass of Lynchburg lemonade.

*Linda Roy is a writer and musician living in New Jersey with her husband and two boys. Her blog* <u>elleroy was here</u> *is a mix of humor and music she refers to as "funny with a soundtrack". She was named a 2014 BlogHer Voice of the Year for humor and has co-authored several anthologies. She is a regular contributor at* The Huffington Post *and* Humor Outcasts *and her work has been featured at Scary Mommy,* In the Powder Room, Erma Bombeck Writers' Workshop, BlogHer, Mamapedia, BonBon Break, Midlife Boulevard, Aiming Low, *and* The Weeklings.

# OH, NO HE DIDN'T

## Stephanie Marsh

Years ago, when my husband and I still had lives before we were married with three children, we were a little wild. You would never know it seeing us now. He is an upstanding member of the community and the best father my children could ask for. As a husband he loves me unconditionally, accepting my anxiety and depression as nothing more than a hiccup in our lives. He cares for me and our children in a way I find simply amazing. These days, we are in bed by 9:00 p.m. and up at 6:00 a.m. to get the kids off to school. We attend school plays, volunteer at charity events, and sponsor ball teams in our hometown.

We are no longer the people we were when this story took place. (He made me tell you that.) The time I'm talking about, we were in our early twenties and as silly and carefree as only twenty-year-olds can be. He played in a band and I went to all of his shows, which were often and frequently out of control. Think heavy metal, heavy drinking, and partying until daylight. Ah, those were the days.

Generally, I would fall out first because of my unbelievably low tolerance for alcohol. This night though, my husband outdid himself. His band opened for one of his favorite bands and he celebrated all night long. People were buying him shots, he was buying himself shots, and by the end of the night he didn't even know where he was—and I didn't know how he was still standing.

He was so drunk that I had to load his equipment for him. If you have ever known a musician, you might know what a big deal this is. In all the years we had been together, I had never, ever touched his drum set. He had never left a gig without breaking it down and packing it up as gently as if it were his child. So while he stood there and made an ass of himself—I mean, stood there and gestured grandly while making a meaningful speech laced with "I love you man" and lots of curse words—I packed up his shit.

After I had everything loaded safely into the back of our car, I called a cab. There was no way either of us was driving anywhere, even the short distance to our motel, and walking there was out because he couldn't even stand up straight.

Once the cabbie got us to the motel, I managed to get him to the room and into the bed. He was asleep in seconds and I was asleep not much later.

Sometime during the night, I felt something tickling my face. I brushed it off and tried to go back to sleep, but it got worse until, in the confusion of sleepiness, I decided that it must be raining on me. I woke up fully expecting to be outside in a storm. Instead, I found myself on a bed in a hotel room with a jackass.

I opened my eyes and found my loving husband on his knees in the bed, dick out, urinating on his pillow. With dawning horror, I watched the urine hit the pillow and splash about the bed. It took me a moment to digest the fact he had pretty much just pissed on my face.

I jumped up off the bed and yelled, "What the fuck!?"

He slowly turned his head toward me and gave me this look as if he didn't know how I had the audacity to speak to him while he was clearly otherwise occupied. He would later tell me that he dreamt I had followed him into the men's room.

I obviously wasn't going to get any sense out of him so I left him there and went to frantically scrub my face and wash my hair. I was furious.

I came back out of the bathroom with some choice words for him and found him passed back out, face down. On his pillow. Which he had just thoroughly soaked with his own urine.

I decided he had punished himself enough for the moment, though he didn't know it yet, and proceeded to curl up in a little ball at the foot of the bed, shaking my head, still not believing what had just happened.

The next morning, he woke me up and had no idea what he had done. He was all, "Hey, baby, how *you* doin'?" and I was all, "Listen, asshole, you pissed on my face last night."

Despite all this, I ended up marrying the man and he has supported me through all the ups and downs that have come with living with my depression and anxiety. He's never pissed on me again and I have made a concerted effort to not piss on his dreams either—even if they do take me outside my comfort zone every now and then.


*Stephanie Marsh likes words and suspects she would like sanity, but really has no way of knowing. She can be reasonable, but not often. You can find her on her blog, We Don't Chew Glass, and in the soon to be released anthology,* Adventures in Potty Training and Other Bathroom Mishaps.

# WHEN THE DOCTOR SAYS, "YOU'RE BIPOLAR"

## Jessica Azar

"I know what's wrong with you," the doctor said as she folded her hands behind her head. "You're bipolar. You have bipolar disorder, type II. That's why the antidepressants you've been taking work great for a while, then just stop working. Your body chemistry needs a mood stabilizer to temper the antidepressant, or you'll have too much serotonin. This shoots you up, and then you crash." It was like a bomb had been detonated, leaving me in jagged pieces of confusing emotions.

I sat there in silence, then pasted a well-practiced smile on my face, the mask that's helped me coast publicly through long periods of misery and said, "Well it's good to know why the meds quit working. What's the difference between bipolar and bipolar II?"

She answered me with a patient, though somewhat condescending, tone. "As a bipolar II patient, you won't typically experience the wild manias that are a hallmark of bipolar disorder. Manias are where one goes on alcohol binges, spending sprees, or engages in other risky behaviors. You instead have hypomania, which includes severe irritability, insomnia, pressured speech, and other milder, but still invasive symptoms. A hypomanic episode usually precedes a plunge into deep depression. As a bipolar II patient, these depressive episodes are more severe than those of someone with classic bipolar disorder." She paused a second and looked at me meaningfully, then said, "That's why a higher suicide rate is associated with bipolar II. The depressions are more frequent and can be harder to emerge from."

*Higher suicide rates? More severe depressions? I don't even experience the* woohoo *of classic manias? I can't even have the "more enjoyable" variety of this mess?* I thought to myself. Even the "ups" I endured were mentally oppressive and hellish. I now know that manias can be catastrophically destructive to a person's life, but at this point I was in shock and feeling cheated in a myriad of ways.

"Now what do I do? Where do I go from here?" I said with a forced, yet believable cheerfulness.

I was somewhat relieved to hear that there was a name for the endless roller coaster of moods and emotions that had ruled my life for so long, but it fueled my anxiety at the same time. I could practically hear the *clank* of the prison bars coming down around me, because being imprisoned is what it felt like. From voracious prior research, I knew that bipolar is incurable. It's a life sentence. I also knew there are ways to manage symptoms, but there is no "one size fits all" treatment for bipolar disorder, and tons of variables to consider. My shoulders struggled against the weight of the news. They sagged under the knowledge that managing my symptoms could be like a part-time job, depending on my needs. It was overwhelming.

"It's a good thing that you already have children, because having more isn't a wise choice for you now that you know what you're up against. Pregnancy and bipolar don't go together. You know how horribly you felt after both of your sons' deliveries? That can actually get worse with subsequent births," the doctor said, very matter-of-factly.

My mind jolted with the realization that I did, in fact, have two very young kids (my sons were barely two years old and ten months old at this point in time) and my diagnosis would affect them. What if I couldn't hold it all together? What if I crumbled beneath the demands of being a mother and trying to keep my illness in check? And I was *horrified* at the thought of not being able to safely (in terms of my sanity) have more children. I always had dreamed of having four kids. While I was grateful for my sons, her statement felt like a slap in the face and a kick in the heart. "So I can't have any more children?" I asked evenly, hiding my horror.

As she removed her glasses, she said, "As we discussed, your postpartum depression was severe after your oldest son's birth, and also bad following your younger son's birth. You would have to go off of all of your mental health medicines at the first sign of pregnancy, and that within itself can be catastrophic. Why would you want to put yourself and everyone else through that hell? It's just not worth it."

I was stunned. She was rebuking me for even entertaining the thought of additional children. I felt like I was being treated like a child or someone who couldn't control any aspect of her behavior. My life plans were being laid out before me in relation to my new "limitations" and it felt as if my control over my own destiny was being repossessed. Inside my head a tiny voice screamed through the brain fog of depression, "This cannot be right! You know yourself. Your life is not over. You are still in control of yourself."

She wrote out prescriptions for a higher dosage of my current antidepressant, an anti-anxiety medication, and a mood stabilizer. Part of me was excited about the prospect of feeling better, emerging from the isolating mental fog that had surrounded me for so long, and actually enjoying my kids for once. Another part of me was scared the medicines would make things worse. The doctor had warned me of that possibility, and also cautioned me I would probably never feel great, but that we were going for "good enough." Good enough to function sanely, good enough to make it from one day to the next, good enough to not burden the lives of my family with my symptoms. This didn't sit well with me, because I'm not the type of person who accepts "good enough" for myself. I'm a highly driven, goal-oriented individual—that is, when I'm not in the pits of the hell of depression. I knew I would need to explore accompanying treatment options to enable myself to surpass the "good enough" range of functioning; I had dreams to pursue and a life to live.

At that moment, I began to realize that while managing bipolar II was not going to be easy, doing my best to do so was the key to living out an amazingly fulfilling life. I already had what I needed to truly survive inside of me: my determination, faith in God, and a thirst for the knowledge to find accompanying treatments. Making use of those has taken me far, and six years after being diagnosed (and successfully having two more children) my life isn't always easy, but I wouldn't trade it. Using those internal resources has shown me that changes in diet, medications, and exercise, as well as a good support system, are key. In some ways, the feeling of being told I have bipolar disorder has fueled my drive to do things I might not have attempted otherwise, like running a marathon (I discovered that running helps my symptoms) or being published (writing is therapy and allows my creativity to flow). It also inspires me to be an even better mother than I ever dreamed I could.

I have bipolar, and I'm learning that it's not such a horrible thing after all.

*Jessica Azar is a wife and stay-at-home mother to four young children and writes the popular blog Herd Management. She is a NickMom Ambassador,*

NickMom *writer,* Huffington Post *blogger, and* POPSUGAR *Select Blogger. Her writing has been featured on* Huffington Post Parents, Huffington Post Entertainment, BLUNTMoms, POPSUGAR, Venn Magazine *and other websites, and has essays in other published anthologies. When she's not writing, Jessica goes running and drinks single malt scotch to soothe her kid-rattled nerves.*

# AM I GOOD ENOUGH?

## Joy Hedding

I t's funny how depression messes with your mind, your perception, and your reality. Actually it's not funny at all. It's awful.

I look at my life from the outside and it is an amazing life, filled with beauty and blessings. There is a house filled with love and family on a street in suburban America. The table is set with food, a paycheck arrives regularly, and there are no shortages of friends. I live the American Dream.

But there is more you don't see. There is depression with an overabundance of anxiety. I've just put on a pair of glasses meant for someone with very different eyes.

⋑⋐⋑⋐

I had a great marriage, a healthy son, a job I was good at that paid well. I had a beautiful home and a loving family. It was all I had dreamed of, but it was tainted.

In depression, I was failure at everything I touched. I was a conductor of all things terrible. I didn't want to be near or associate myself with anything for fear of causing it ruin.

After having my first child, I struggled to return to my pre-pregnancy weight—a challenge faced by many women. I couldn't get my head around the fact an 8-plus-pound baby left my body with ten pounds more to lose. I was covered in tiger stripes from my breasts to my thighs, from front to back. I believed my husband couldn't possibly be happy with the fat woman I had become after having our baby. How could he possibly look at me and be attracted?

Depression convinced me he would be so much better off with another woman. A woman who was *more*, who could cook meals and keep a house clean. A woman who could do the laundry and not fall asleep at 8:00 p.m. A woman who didn't have to drive so far to work, so she would be home more and be more of a mother. This is what I believed.

Time passed and I remained trapped in my depressed mind. Like any parent, I worried about every bump, bruise, sneeze, or sniffle my child experienced. However, anxiety turned the level of worry to one of obsession. For example, my son needed glasses at age two. My natural reaction was that I had caused his eyesight problems because I developed diabetes during his pregnancy. Maybe it was because I failed to deliver him vaginally and had a c-section. My mind invented possibilities of what I did wrong to cause him to need glasses. I kept thinking he would be so much better off with a new mama, one who wasn't so terrible.

I was successful at my job. I was a bright young woman with a degree in applied mathematics working in a field few women braved. I was advancing quickly; I was promoted in under two years with the company, and received a thirty percent pay raise in the same period. Yet my mind wouldn't rest; it kept telling me I could do more. I could be better. I could understand at a higher level the inner workings of whatever system I was designing training programs for. I could teach classes in a more efficient style. I was sure someone else could do this better. I was trapped in a crazy cycle—do more, do better, not enough. Repeat.

Looking back, I realize depression and anxiety took a prominent role when my firstborn was little, right after he was born. I should have been happy. I was, but not like a new parent should be. I cried constantly. I didn't know why. Why was I not happy? Is this the dreaded "baby blues?" But I pushed forward and after a few months I fell into a routine, an obsessive routine.

I went to bed each evening sure he was going to die from SIDS. I checked on him upwards of ten times a night to ensure he was breathing. I checked to make sure he was on his back, that he didn't have any suffocation hazards. I checked throughout the evening to make sure no one had taken him. My anxiety had no limits or boundaries.

I would rise at 4:00 a.m. to pump because I was *obsessed* with my son having only breast milk. That was the one thing I was good at and that only I could do, but still the worries never rested. I punished myself for drinking a Diet Pepsi. I was certain I was doing him harm from ingesting caffeine. I would pump and dump twelve ounces every day lest I cause damage to his developing brain and body. After pumping two bottles worth of milk I would feed him. I made sure he made eye contact with me and made sure he smiled. The fight to treat autism early had begun in earnest through magazine campaigns the year before he was born. Public awareness was on the rise and I *had* to check every day for signs he was or was not on the spectrum.

By 5:15 a.m. I would be out the door for work. It was a 50-minute drive with little or no traffic. Most days it took me a just over an hour, each way. And every day as I passed a building only a mile from our home I punished myself; I had a job offer from that company and I choose this one far from home. How could I be so stupid?

I worked like a crazy person. Often eating my lunch at my desk. Who would want to hang out with me? Why would anyone want to hear my voice? Ever? Even when teaching my classes I hated the sound my voice made.

I would leave the office as soon as I could. But even that isn't technically true—I could only leave work when I felt like I'd finally done enough. I often stayed late and worked longer just to do what I thought was required of someone "like me."

At home my husband cooked dinner. He picked our son up from daycare. He played with him. He was such a good dad. I was just ruining everything by ... being. And so I looked for an escape.

I found excuses to go places across the river from our house. I thought about driving my car off a nearby bridge, but then at the last minute I'd chicken out and bring my son. I knew I would never hurt my child. I thought I was being a coward because I couldn't go through with it. I knew if I brought him to the store located across the river from our house I would bring him home. I would have to keep living another day. He was my savior.

⟫⟪

I'm thankful every day I was a chicken. I've come to realize I was deep in the throws of depression. I lived my life and hid it well. Many people had no idea how messed up inside I was, or how much I struggled.

I finally came out of the fog of anxiety and depression I was living in during the middle of my second pregnancy. I felt the sun and I longed for the day to start. Unfortunately, I had a false sense of security. My mind betrayed me when I delivered my second child. The depression and anxiety were even worse this time but I knew to seek help; I couldn't go through that hell again.

My OBGYN at the time underestimated the depth of my illness when he put me on an anxiety med for only three months. When I asked for a refill he counseled, "You should be better." I thought he was right, I rationalized that he should know he was the doctor. I didn't speak up, I didn't explain my concerns, and I didn't say anything. I was left with no choice but to stop taking the medicine cold turkey. I spiraled out of control.

The perfect storm was brewing.

I was no longer working outside the home. I had two small children and spent a lot of time alone. I was compulsive about doing everything right. I wanted to be the perfect mother. We had a letter of the day, a color of the day, and new words to work on each morning and afternoon. There was no television for my babies because it was bad for them, and if I allowed them to have anything bad for them then I was bad. I was dedicated to making all their baby food versus buying it, but I couldn't keep up with the other tasks I needed to complete. The house was a disaster, nothing was put away, and I was behind on laundry. If I couldn't get *everything* done then I wasn't getting *anything* done. I was failing at life, again. I couldn't keep up with the demands I created for myself.

And then a wonderful thing happened: I had a minor car incident. I went home and bawled incessantly for ten hours. I made my husband drive me back out to the area to make sure the damage I did didn't cause an accident that killed someone. When I demanded he take me back to the scene of my accident he finally realized my issues were bigger than he thought. That day he told me, "It's time to see someone." My husband stood by me through all of this—every day—for many years. He never wavered even when I thought he should. Without him, I don't know where I'd be. Or if I'd still ... be.

That appointment began a 12-year journey I am still on today. I found a doctor who heard me. She started me on a new prescription—one that worked for me this time. I also saw a therapist for a short while but she wasn't a good fit for me. I retreated further and further into myself after failing with my therapist. I didn't know enough or have enough confidence to seek another therapist and took all she said as gospel. In hindsight, I now know the problem wasn't with me; the two of us did not work well together.

Shortly after my failed counseling sessions, our family moved. I found another great doctor and an amazing therapist. It took a lot of work to get to the place where I can say:

I'm a good person.

I'm a good wife.

I'm a great mother.

I'm not conceited. It's still hard for me to type those words. It's hard to not hit backspace and erase "great" and type "okay." But in my heart, I know I'm a great mom. I just have to remind myself.

I do my best. And finally ... my best is good enough.

*Joy, aka Evil Joy, is wife to one Dr. Evil and mother to four children she lovingly refers to as spawn. Joy started blogging in late 2011 as a way to communicate with her family and friends about an illness her family experienced and continues to blog about life as she sees fit. She loves to read, run, snowboard, and spend time running her spawn to all of their various activities – all of which she's been known to blog about. Frequently funny, always honest, and occasionally serious Joy writes about everything from dealing with messy teenagers to living life with depression, anxiety and PTSD on her blog* Evil Joy Speaks.

# HAVE FUN WITH YOUR MENTAL ILLNESS!

## Nicole Leigh Shaw

When I was stressed out by my upcoming wedding, out-of-state move, and first home purchase, which were all slated to happen within a two-week period, my mental state was in chaos. Before I realized that my anxiety and depression were out of control, I did what any irrational, emotionally explosive person would do: I threw a cup of iced tea at a Burger King worker. Oh you should've heard the laughter of everyone in the restaurant! (Except the guy wearing my large cup of iced tea and myself, beset as I was by unmitigated rage, of course.) One gal's hissy fit is a Burger King patron's afternoon comedy show!

The back story is thin, I'm afraid. I ordered a sandwich. I waited a long time, by typical fast food standards. Then, when I thought my food was finally arriving, they gave my sandwich—my sandwich!—to some *employee*.

There was a moment, right before I threw my beverage at the back of a cashier, which illustrates the level of commitment to which only the batshit crazy can cling. I was screaming for a refund and coaching the young man at the register in the finer points of currency calculations, saying things like, "You do know how to add, right?" when I heard the cashier to his right say, "We need security at the counter." I'd elevated the terror level to hot pink: Crazy Bitch Ordering a Burger. He'd called the rest stop security officers on me! This after making me wait seven, maybe eight minutes for a hamburger! How *dare* he?

The cashier turned away, assuming, I imagine, that security would take his spot as "guy getting tongue-lashing from a hangry (hungry and angry) person." This was my chance to take a deep breath and relax. In the movie of my life, this was the slow-mo moment when there'd be a voice over, the main character (me) revealing to the audience that this moment mattered, and that good choices would be made.

My life, however, is not a movie. I took the top off of my large beverage and flung the contents at the back of the cashier, shouting, "Don't you turn your back on me!" (Hot tip: never turn your back on a psycho.)

Silver lining: I was not arrested.

Other silver lining: In reflecting on this incident, I learned something I will share with you. It's call self-diagnosis. I don't mean in the larger sense that you should try to be your own doctor, just that some of our actions can tell us a lot about our bigger issues. Just like the itch that's really eczema, your blues could really be moderate depression. Be aware of what may *really* be going on with you, below the surface.

I know many people have trouble seeing mental illness or their "crazy" in this light, but it's helped me so much in two important ways:

First of all, I live my life and "crazy" out in the open. I feel compelled to divest myself of my mistakes and cop to my oddities. I've never been accused of having a shy and retiring nature and I'm as likely to give a stranger the time as I am to give her my life story. It's like confession, good for my soul. It's also a great way to ruin a date, but somehow I still wound up married.

Second, I use my sense of humor to my advantage. I don't let trifling things like propriety or a sense of boundaries stop me from laughing. For instance, when my father died my grandfather discovered his stash of pot as we were cleaning out Dad's apartment. "Do you want your father's drug paraphernalia?" he'd asked me. When your seventy-year-old grandfather asks you, very sincerely, if you want to keep your dead father's doobage, you need to laugh. Do it even if you feel like bawling your eyes out from grief and the fog of depression is closing in on you; it's central to surviving and thriving.

Look, I know I'm not necessarily the same brand of whacko as my fellow whackos, but I do know this: if you can't talk about it, you can't deal with it, and if you can't deal with it, you'll never appreciate exactly how funny it is. In every insane moment, whether it's manically shopping for your fifty-seventh pair of socks on a manic bipolar high, or breathing through an anxiety attack because you can't bring yourself to pee in a public restroom but you really have to go, realize that you'll emerge from this moment stronger. When rational, stable thinking has found its way back into your mind, you will be able to laugh about these idiosyncrasies, and remember that those moments make the best stories and keep life from being dull. Do your best to find the funny in your crazy, because it lets the sorrow out as sure as it lets the sanity in.

*Nicole Leigh Shaw lives by the motto that all four of her kids are still breathing. Award, please. You can find her blogging on her site, Nicole Leigh Shaw, where she's embarrassed her mother many, many times.*

# EPILOGUE
## Dr. Margaret Rutherford

There is nothing inherently funny about mental illness.

Like anything that has the capacity to sabotage the quality of your life—to change the manner in which you think of yourself, or make you fear how others will perceive you—it's not humorous. It can be scary. Daunting. Confusing. Paralyzing.

It's not pleasant to be unable to predict what your mood is likely to be in the next two hours. It's not affirming to want to go to your daughter's basketball game and know that the way-too-strong adrenaline rush you will feel as soon as you are among the crowd will make you shake and fight the impulse to flee.

It's not a confidence-builder that you wrestle with the urge to throw up after a meal. Or clean the bathtub with a toothbrush every night. Or struggle to not watch more porn. Or gamble. Or drink.

None of that is amusing.

During my graduate school training, I worked at Parkland Hospital's psychiatric emergency center in Dallas. I saw a lot of people who were acutely ill. I distinctly remember a woman who came in. She was about forty-five years old. Had huge muscles in her arms and legs. Soft-spoken. Miserable.

She described a strange compulsion to move all of her furniture out of her home, place it in her yard, and put it back. Every day. Come rain or shine. These activities consumed her otherwise fairly normal existence.

I remember what she said as she laughed. "I have even tried working for a moving company. It helped some. But when I got home, I still had the need to pick up a chair. Out it went."

What did her attempt at humor about her situation tell me about her? First, she recognized that hers was a more unique symptom. (I have never met anyone else with that particular compulsion.) More importantly, it reflected her ability to detach herself, even for a moment, from the actual pain of her life.

That is what is termed in the world of psychology as "ego strength". The ability for self-care. To be able to maintain a sense of vitality. Use good decision-making. Adapt. Compartmentalize pain.

It's that part of you that can muster the strength to not act on every thought or emotion and soothe yourself through hurt or trouble. Will yourself to do other things that are difficult to accomplish.

Sometimes that involves laughing.

This particular patient was using whatever she could find "funny" in her situation to try to cope. To handle what life had handed her. She was fighting feeling defeated by compulsions that ate up her day and were ruinous to the enjoyment of her life. But she was still fighting. She was still searching for help.

Seeing the humor in her situation gave her something to have control over. Something she could do in that moment to ease her pain.

Kay Jamison, a renowned expert on bipolar disorder, is doing something similar:

*"But money spent while manic doesn't fit into the Internal Revenue Service concept of medical expense or business loss. So after mania, when most depressed, you're given excellent reason to be even more so."*— Kay Redfield Jamison, An Unquiet Mind: A Memoir of Moods and Madness

Not funny when you take her words literally. Think about the actual consequence of severe, impulsive, manic over-spending. But she is allowing herself to recognize the irony of the situation. At least smile about something.

Laughter—seeing the humor in a situation, however ironically— gives you a sense of control.

Many of the authors you have just read—or, if you like to read the end of a book first, you are *about* to read—have done just that. Looked for what was funny or poignant in their lives. Some wrote pieces that were informative. Some were reeling with intensity and pain.

All gave me hope. Hope that we are no longer hiding. Hope that our culture is ready to understand more about mental illness. Talk more openly. Be compassionate.

What that also means is that, with less stigma, maybe … just maybe … more people will get the treatment they need.

That would be astonishingly wonderful.

I thought of my patients while reading this manuscript. Some stride into my waiting room. Write on their Facebook page that they are in therapy. Couldn't care less whether or not someone sees them walk in my door. Talk to their friends and family about what we discuss.

Others wait until the last minute to enter. Make sure the person who is before them leaves before they covertly make their way in. I am not allowed to call them at work. Maybe they don't even want statements sent to their home.

Their mental and emotional struggles are shameful to them. They remain nervous of what others will think of them.

Books like this anthology are meant to dispel this stigma. Each of the stories has been written by a well-respected blogger or author, and is dealing with mental illness of one form or another.

You have probably read this book because you yourself experience mental illness, or someone you love does.

All of these writers opened up their lives for you to know you are not alone.

That it is more than okay to talk about what you are going through. And laugh at what you can.

Mental illness can be demoralizing. It can wring from your spirit the sense that your life can be good and productive. But when you can laugh, even if there is a tear in your eye, you are moving through those feelings.

I know when I hear a patient laugh—tell me they enjoyed a joke or a text, or just smile a bit as they talk—they are getting better. They may have been talking about killing themselves a month ago. But the lights are beginning to come back on.

Hope is being aroused from a long sleep.

That doesn't mean that the next day, or the next hour, they will be able to find that glimmer.

But every time we can, we gain ground. Ground that's not lost simply because the giggle goes away. It has had an impact.

I laugh a lot. And I have had my fair share of panic attacks. Throw in some time spent with anorexia and a couple of dates with depression...Let's just say I have learned about managing symptoms.

If we can laugh, we can ease that moment. Get perspective. Take a little control.

And enjoy what we can about the life we have been given.

*Dr. Margaret Rutherford is a clinical psychologist who has been practicing in Fayetteville, Arkansas. Her writing from her website, http://drmargaretrutherford.com is featured on the Huffington Post, Boomeon, Midlife Boulevard, BetterAfter50 and others. She has treated hundreds of patients with depression, anxiety, trauma and personality disorders over the last 20 years. She received the 2009 Arkansas Psychological Association's Private Practitioner of the Year award and is an Adjunct Professor of Psychiatry at the University of Arkansas Medical School.  She has authored an eBook,* "Seven Commandments of Good Therapy", *which is available on her website.*

# DISCLAIMER

The Surviving Mental Illness Through Humor anthology's sole purpose is to share personal stories the individual authors have experienced. This book does not purpose to diagnose, recommend, approve or disprove any mental illnesses. This book is not responsible for any medical claims, or actions. The Surviving Mental Illness Through Humor anthology is primarily a source of community amongst those who suffer from mental illness. The experiences of all of the authors are individual to them, and by no means should be interpreted to be a reason to seek or not to seek any medical guidance or intervention. All contributors hope that if you are in need or require any assistance you will immediately seek a trained medical professional.

Furthermore, by trade the contributors are writers and authors. We have all found this to be a therapeutic means of handling our own illnesses, and hope that you will find what works for you on your journey.

Thank you for taking the time to read this anthology of heartfelt and hysterical pieces by some of the bravest writers we know.

Alyson Herzig and Jessica Azar

# SMITH CONTRIBUTOR CHARITY SELECTIONS

Al-Anon *(Kristen Kelley)*
The Al-Anon Family Groups are a fellowship of relatives and friends of alcoholics who share their experience, strength, and hope in order to solve their common problems. We believe alcoholism is a family illness and that changed attitudes can aid recovery.

ALS Support *(Marcia Kester Doyle)*
Leading the fight to treat and cure ALS through global research and nationwide advocacy while also empowering people with Lou Gehrig's Disease and their families to live fuller lives by providing them with compassionate care and support.

American Foundation for Suicide Prevention *(Stephanie Marsh, Kathryn Leehane)*
We fund research, create educational programs, advocate for public policy, support survivors of suicide loss, and are a leader in the fight against suicide.

Angel of Hope Memorial Garden *(Noelle Elliott)*
The Angel of Hope Memorial Garden is created to be a place of reflection and remembrance for all who have lost a child.

ASPCA *(Katie Hiener)*
We believe that animals are entitled to kind and respectful treatment at the hands of humans, and must be protected under the law.

Born Free *(Zoe Lewis)*
Born Free takes action worldwide to protect threatened species and stop individual animal suffering. Born Free believes wildlife belongs in the wild and works to phase out zoos. We rescue animals from lives of misery in tiny cages and give them lifetime care.

Canadian Mental Health Association *(Leighann Adams)*
Canadian Mental Health Association promotes the mental health of all and supports the resilience and recovery of people experiencing mental illness. The CMHA accomplishes this mission through advocacy, education, research and service.

Canadian Mental Health Association of Windsor-Essex County *(Kimberly Morand)*
We teach how to take care of your mental health through the education of facts about mental illness, offering solutions for yourself or others.

Capital Area United Way *(Audrey Hayworth)*
To improve lives by leveraging partnerships in our community to advance the common good through education, income stability, and healthy living.

Every Mother Counts *(Michelle Matthews)*

EMC is dedicated to making pregnancy and childbirth safe for every mother. We raise funds to support maternal health programs around the world.

Footprints Ministry *(Jessica Azar)*
The Ultimate Goal of Footprints Ministry is to share the love of Christ with NICU families in such a way that each and every person is strengthened, comforted, and reminded that they are not alone on their NICU journey.

Hamilton Center *(Veronica Leigh)*
Hamilton Center is a regional behavioral health system serving central and west central Indiana. We are "building hope and changing lives" through a broad array of behavioral health services.

Kick Cancer Movement *(Joy Hedding)*
KICKcancER is dedicated to helping families affected by childhood cancer THRIVE. Our goal is to empower through education— teaching the importance of *real food, real health,* and how to implement it into *real life*—both during and after treatment.

March of Dimes *(Tricia Stream)*
We help moms have full-term pregnancies and research the problems that threaten the health of babies.

Miscarriage Association *(Lauren B. Stevens)*
The Miscarriage Association acknowledges the distress associated with pregnancy loss and strives to make a positive difference to those that are affected.

NAMI (National Alliance of Mental Illness) *(Nicole Knepper, Barbara Blank, Jenn Rian)*

NAMI, the National Alliance on Mental Illness, is the nation's largest grassroots mental health organization dedicated to building better lives for the millions of Americans affected by mental illness.

NAMI Indiana *(Abby Heugel, Nicole Leigh Shaw)*

NAMI Lane County *(Sherry Vondy Beaver)*

NAMI Maine *(Lynn Shattuck)*

NAMI New Jersey *(Linda Roy)*

National Eating Disorders Association *(Carrie Groves)*
NEDA supports individuals and families affected by eating disorders, and serves as a catalyst for prevention, cures and access to quality care.

Nelson House *(Tammy Rutledge)*
Nelson House exists to provide safety for women and children who are being abused and to work with other groups and individuals toward ending violence against all women.

Northern Virginia Mental Health *(Kathleen Gordon)*
Often people receiving mental health services have additional needs for goods and services for which there is no personal or other funding. The client and his or her clinician can apply for NVMHF funds to help the client reach treatment goals.

Northwest Arkansas Free Health Clinic (Dr. Margaret Rutherford)
NWAFHC Provides health care to low-income individuals regardless of their ability to pay.

Please Live *(Andrea Keeney)*

The purpose and mission of Please Live shall be to promote help, welfare, and healing of at-risk teenage and college age students by providing educational and referral services to students, parents, and community members regarding depression, self-injury, and similar mental health issues which may lead to suicide and other unproductive life outcomes.

Postpartum Education and Support North Carolina *(Leigh Baker)*
PESNC is an organization dedicated to the emotional wellness of mothers. We offer support for mothers and their families, provide resources for health care providers, and heighten public awareness of perinatal mood disorders.

Rape, Abuse, Incest National Network *(Lea Grover)*
The nation's largest anti-sexual violence organization and was named one of "America's 100 Best Charities" by Worth magazine. RAINN created and operates the National Sexual Assault Hotline (800.656. HOPE and online.rainn.org) in partnership with more than 1,100 local rape crisis centers across the country.

St. Margaret's House *(Alyson Herzig)*
St. Margaret's House improves the lives of women and children by providing individual attention to their immediate needs, breaking the bonds of isolation and helping them acquire skills to better their lives. Through a philosophy of shared ownership in St. Margaret's House, guests become empowered by participating in planning and decision making.

# CALL FOR SUBMISSIONS

Do you have a story to tell? Do you or a loved one suffer from mental illness? Come join the fight to end the stigma and submit your story to the next book in the series of Surviving Mental Illness Through Humor. We are looking for first person stories that detail the depths of your illness, or a humorous tale that has your mental illness woven into it. To find more information please go to the Surviving Mental Illness website and learn how to submit to our next volume. Together we can change the world and laugh stigma into submission.

Made in the USA
Charleston, SC
07 April 2015